Career Skills for Doctors

Charalambos Panayiotou Charalambous

Career Skills for Doctors

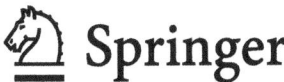 Springer

Charalambos Panayiotou Charalambous,
BSc, MBChB, MSc, MD, FRCS (Orth)
Department of Trauma and Orthopaedics
Blackpool Victoria Hospital
Blackpool
UK

The sketches (figures) included in this article were drawn by Robert Brownlow, commissioned by CP Charalambous. The copyright is held by CP Charalambous.

ISBN 978-3-319-13478-9   ISBN 978-3-319-13479-6   (eBook)
DOI 10.1007/978-3-319-13479-6
Springer Cham Heidelberg New York Dordrecht London

Library of Congress Control Number: 2014960062

Printed on acid-free paper

Springer is part of Springer Science+Business Media (www.springer.com)

I dedicate this book to my parents and to all my special teachers and trainers

Foreword I

The ability of a healthcare provider to function optimally requires a vast set of skills, knowledge, behaviours and attitudes many of which are not inherent, not taught overtly, and are often acquired as part of the training and maturation experience. The importance of inclusiveness of the multi-professional and multi-disciplinary team in optimizing patient outcomes should be obvious. The value and benefit of a simple, yet comprehensive resource that addresses many of the questions and concerns of the young practitioner is a welcome addition to all.

This new book *Career Skills for Doctors* intends to provide advice and counsel for many of the questions and concerns not formally addressed in our curricula. This text, created by a successful practicing surgeon in England, is a collection of broad yet practical topics that will apply to all practitioners in Medicine, especially physicians. The text provides personal guidance about basic skills in communication and teamwork, prioritization, organization and efficiency. The text serves as a rich resource for reflection and implementation of new skills by providing a wide array of examples and by using questions and simple statements to direct improvement efforts. Importantly, the book also includes sections on self-evaluation of your current practices (audit), and how to approach research, presentations, and publication as well as principles of learning and teaching. While the book is obviously written and applies to the British training schema, the lessons included are universally applicable with the minor translation of terms such as post and attachment with residency program.

This book is useful to those who are healthcare students, beginning doctors who would benefit from this comprehensive review of the fundamental knowledge or skills that are needed in today's world. Further this book serves as an opportunity for those who may already have completed their training to re-examine their practices and consider if they have optimized the incorporation and functioning of many of the skills included in this book. The book is intended to serve as a single resource for the developing healthcare practitioner providing numerous examples, detailed discussion of each topic, and selected references for further query when needed. The book is well organized into sections: it can be read in one sitting, or sections can be accessed as the need arises, whether it is as a student approaches the wards for the first time, or when the trainee is now looking for their first position. The reader will want to read and reread many of the sections several times. The use of quotations throughout adds charm and emphasis to each section. When in the age of innumerable texts and electronic data sources this book serves as a compendium of "how to" topics as single text and its comprehensiveness is perhaps its greatest strength.

Students will find this manual helpful in the practical advice you will gain about how to conduct yourself and how to think about your role in a team. Young trainees will find the topics related to productivity essential. Aspiring academics will find this book helpful in understanding the scope of practice, what may be expected in their future, and how they may go about teaching, presentations, and research. Any provider will want to ensure they are familiar with and have optimized all of the topics in this book. The author should be commended for taking on, and articulately accomplishing, such a timely and valuable task. While this book is clearly titled and directed toward physicians, this is really essential reading for all healthcare providers.

Pamela A. Lipsett, MD, MHPE, FCCM
Warfiled M. Firor Endowed Professorship
Professor of Surgery, Anesthesiology
Critical Care Medicine, and Nursing
Johns Hopkins Schools of Medicine and Nursing
Baltimore, MD, USA

Foreword II

"Now what do I do?" This is often the cry of the inexperienced doctor. This book provides a clear guidance through the many pitfalls, minefields, administrative swamps and other impedimenta that seem to beset the doctor in their first jobs and then in their second, third and so on. At each level there always appears to be problems with organisation, problems with administration and problems with just finding the basic time to do the job properly.

It is clear from the text that the author has appreciated that Medicine is not a job, it is a vocation. It is a way of life, it is all encompassing and, having such a text to be able to put your thoughts into the right context and to perform the right actions at the right time, does require an inner organisation which is helped enormously by this book.

It is useful to remember the Latin proverb which says, *"the average man learns by his own mistakes, the wise man by other's mistakes and the fool by nobody's mistakes"*. I would recommend you read this book and use it as an aide-memoire when you are in need of instant wisdom.

Professor J.K. Stanley
Professor of Hand Surgery
Consultant Hand & Upper Limb Surgeon
Wrightington, USA

Preface

The primary objective of this book is to present skills that a doctor may find helpful in day to day workplace practise and in career progression. The inspiration for this book came from personal experiences at various stages of my career, and through the observations of similar challenges that other doctors faced.

The aim of this book is to present information in an easily readable, succinct way, and break down a vast complex subject into small, manageable sections. An attempt is made to provide the reader with knowledge and information, but also stimulate lateral thinking though repeated, often rhetoric, questioning.

I would like to thank Liz Pope, Associate Editor at Springer, for her invaluable help and advice in the preparation and presentation of this book.

Charalambos Panayiotou Charalambous, BSc, MBChB,
MSc, MD, FRCS (Orth)
Department of Trauma and Orthopaedics
Blackpool Victoria Hospital
Blackpool

School of Medicine and Dentistry
University of Central Lancashire
Preston

Faculty of Medical and Human Sciences
University of Manchester
Manchester, UK

Contents

About the Author

Bambos (short name for Charalambos) studied Medicine at the University of Manchester, UK, and did all his postgraduate Surgical and Orthopaedic training in the North West of England. This training involved posts in both central university hospitals and peripheral district hospitals, which provided an appreciation of different working environments with a variety of organisational and work pattern settings.

Bambos is currently a consultant in Trauma and Orthopaedics at Blackpool Teaching Hospitals NHS Foundation Trust, UK, where he leads and manages his team, providing a busy clinical service.

Bambos is an Honorary Visiting Professor in the School of Medicine and Dentistry at the University of Central Lancashire and also has affiliations with the University of Manchester. Bambos has a keen interest in Medical Education acting as clinical and educational supervisor, also as mentor of multiple junior doctors at various levels of training. He is an enthusiast in clinical research and audit, having extensively published in these areas.

Chapter 1
Introduction

The transition from medical school to being a practicing junior doctor is challenging. It requires knowledge and clinical skills but also the ability to efficiently function in the workplace and be a productive valuable member of the medical and non-medical teams. At the same time gaining essential clinical experience, passing postgraduate exams, under-taking research or audit and publishing become essential for career progression. One soon realises that being a doctor is not just a profession but a way of life.

Medical school training equips with medical knowledge and clinical skills that are essential in formulating a patient diagnosis as well as planning and administering appropriate medical treatment. However, the skills of thriving in the workplace and career progression may not be adequately taught. Such skills have then to be acquired by drawing on personal experiences, observing others, or through trial and error. This may sometimes require multiple trials and many errors.

This book presents some well known skills that can help you improve your day to day workplace performance, be efficient and productive, be an inherent part of the team, shine and impress. At the same time advice is given as to how to prepare for postgraduate exams, develop essential technical skills, apply for the next post, successfully participate in research and audit, publish, manage, lead, teach, and train. This generic guidance can be useful for those aspiring to become a generalist or subspecialty doctor, and may be of value in whichever part of the world you practice in.

The first three chapters of this book concentrate on organisation, communication, and professionalism, skills that form the central core of day to day clinical practise. The latter part of the book concentrates on skills required for those activities that supplement clinical work; skills of postgraduate learning and teaching, carrying out research and audit, presenting and publishing. Skills needed in applying for that sought after post and skills that may help you deal with situations when things have gone wrong, are then presented. The final chapter helps to remind that work life balance and taking care of yourself are paramount in Medicine, as in any other profession.

© Springer International Publishing Switzerland 2015
C. Panayiotou Charalambous, *Career Skills for Doctors*,
DOI 10.1007/978-3-319-13479-6_1

The skills given in this book originate from personal training experiences, from the wisdoms of my senior teachers and trainers, and from supervising and mentoring multiple junior doctors. Much of the material presented is common knowledge or has been previously described, and no claim is made in this book for its originality. Sources of presented material have been credited where possible, and apologies are given if any such source has been omitted. Not everyone will agree with the advice presented, and that is understandable and acceptable.

I hope these skills will be of great use in your professional life, and will guide you through successful medical careers.

Chapter 2
Organisation

Being organised, having a structure and order in what you do, can improve your productivity, and enhance your influence upon your workplace. Being organised may help you stay on top of things in dealing with high volume and complex workload that a doctor's role may entail.

The ability to plan, utilise time efficiently and effectively, prioritise, delegate, foresee (so that you give others the time they need or allow for the un-expected), use to-do lists, and the ability to be systematic, are important skills to develop. These skills are described in this chapter. Leading a ward round requires a combination of such skills, and advice is given as how to bring these together in such an important clinical task.

© Springer International Publishing Switzerland 2015
C. Panayiotou Charalambous, *Career Skills for Doctors*,
DOI 10.1007/978-3-319-13479-6_2

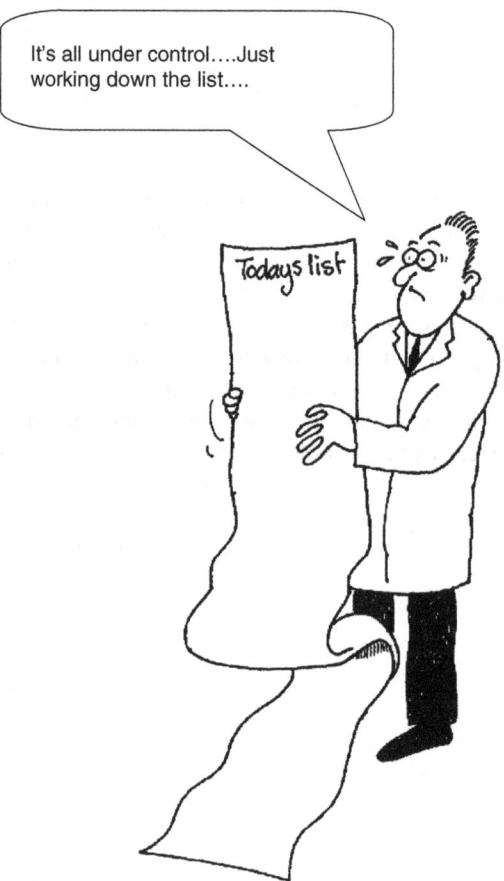

Plan

It takes as much energy to wish as it does to plan

Eleanor Roosevelt [1]

Think of the future, and plan in advance. Think of the next day, next week, next month, next year. What tasks need to be accomplished? What deadlines must be met? What personal commitments must be kept? Think of what is coming and plan how to tackle it. Time spent in planning is time well spent. Planning in advance will let you get organised, juggle things around, avoid last minute rushes, avoid last second panics.

You may plan as how to tackle the various outstanding jobs on your next ward duty, plan in what order to see your on-call referrals, how to revise for the upcoming exams alongside a busy clinical schedule, how to deal with your lengthy list of patients awaiting surgery, how to set up meetings to resolve work issues. You may plan which courses to attend as part of continuous learning, plan for completing all paperwork for your training program assessment, plan for that long awaited holiday, for your wedding, for that weekend break.

Keep an electronic diary, a notebook, a desk calendar, a wall calendar. Note the various upcoming events as you think of them, as they arise. Mark the deadlines, and set warnings for their approach. This will help you think ahead, get organised, and allow you to put a structure to your future ventures.

It may feel like a big transition from medical school days, when many of the yearly events were scheduled by others, when the deadlines were pre-set and known well in advance. It may seem like a life change from university studies, when the main plans were for attending lectures, studying, and passing exams. Some of your activities may still be scheduled by others, by your employer, your supervisors or your trainers. You may have to follow a weekly rota or job plan. You may have to attend clinics, theatres, ward rounds, or be on-call at predefined times. But at last, you can have more flexibility, more control, more influence, in much of your professional life. You can set your goals and the course for the future. Make the most of this by planning in advance.

Be Time Efficient and Time Effective

The bad news is that time flies. The good news is that you are the pilot
Michael Altshuler [1]

You have a set amount of time within which to do various tasks. You have dead-lines to meet, fixed timetables to keep. Not enough time to go round the wards, not much time for your overbooked clinic, limited time for operating, even less time to read and study. The day has so many hours, the week so many days, the year just 12 months. And the tasks are many. Make the most of time, use time efficiently and effectively. How well time is spent is more important than the quantity of time. If you manage your time well, you may be able to accomplish more. The following may help you achieve that:

Allocate time and stick to it
You may allocate time for a meeting, a teaching session, for ringing up a patient's relatives, for seeing each patient in clinic, for completing a ward round, for pre-paring a research presentation, or for having a break. Try and stick to it. Avoid letting time slip by. Try and be one step ahead, rather than a step behind. Keep an eye on the clock, know when to stop, know when to move on.

Allocate tasks according to energy and concentration levels
You may have a multitude of tasks to perform. Some may involve direct clinical care; reviewing or assessing patients, taking bloods, putting a chest drain, insert-ing an arterial line. Some may be administrative tasks; completing discharge summaries, signing letters, ordering tests, completing insurance forms, phar-macy chart refills, entering audit data on a database. Our concentration levels, and alertness, may vary throughout the day [2]. You may be freshest in the morning, more tired and sleepy after a lunch, or as time goes by. You may be an early morning starter, may need a few hours to get going, or may function better later on in the day or night. You may feel more exhausted after assisting in the-atre or after a busy clinic. Try and allocate the most important tasks, those that require the highest alertness, to the time when you feel the best. But still, use the rest of the time in doing those tasks, that can be safely accomplished, even when not at your best.

Minimise empty time
In completing one task you may rely on other staff doing their bit first. Instead of stopping and waiting, leaving that as empty time, try and make use of it. You may consider the following:

- You are doing a ward round, you want to have a look at a patient's wound, you ask the nurse to take the dressings down, but the nurse is busy. Go and do something else, whilst the dressing is taken down. Say you will be back, and do be back on time.
- You are in clinic, you see a patient, and need to review the results of the last blood tests, but these are not in the hospital records. Ask one of your admin-istrative assistants to ring the laboratory to get those results, and try seeing another patient whilst that happens.

- You are a surgeon, you are operating, you know what surgical instrument you will need next. Ask the nurse to get the next instrument ready, before you need it, rather than having to wait for it. The next instrument should be out and in the tray, but on occasions someone may have to go to the store room, to look for it.
- You are doing a ward round in intensive care, you want to insert an arterial line in an un-well patient, ask the staff to get the equipment ready, whilst you continue your ward round and then come back for it.
- You are doing a clinic, some patients may need to have an up to date radiograph in their next clinic visit. You may fill the radiograph request card so it is ready for next time. You save time for patients waiting before sent for the radiograph, and you save yourself time waiting for the patient to return from the radiology department.
- You are in clinic, ensure the staff assisting you, know to bring the next patient into the examination room, whilst you are writing in the notes or dictating a letter for the last patient.
- You just consented and marked, in the ward, the first patient for your surgical list. You are about to set off to theatres at the other end of the hospital. Ring the theatre staff to inform them that the first patient is ready, and that the patient can be sent for. By the time you reach theatres and change in your scrubs, the patient may thus have arrived.

Minimise travel time – Hospitals are huge places, wards are often lengthy. You may have to review patients throughout the hospital, review patients in various bays. You may be on home visits with patients all over town. Choose the best plan to take you smoothly round.

- Avoid running back and forth to the computer to check the blood results or the radiographs of the next patient to be reviewed. Print and carry those, or go through them, before the start of the ward round.
- Carry forms with you to complete investigations requests at the bed site, or make a note of what is needed and fill those at the end of the round.
- Carry with you other essentials, your stethoscope, light torch, reflex hammer, skin marker, according to your duties and specialty, rather than wondering, looking for one around.
- If setting up your own office, your own clinic, your own practise, take travel time into account. Where will patients be seated in clinic? How far do they need to walk before they enter the examination room? Should any patient attending for a wound check be going straight to the dressing room rather than coming first into the consultation room? Where should wards be located in relation to the Emergency Department? Where should theatres be located in relation to the wards?

Limit interruptions

You may want to concentrate on a particular task, but you repeatedly get interrupted. It maybe the ward staff, keep coming up to you with questions, it maybe your pager going off, your phone receiving text messages, your electronic tablet bleeping every time a new email arrives. Try and eliminate any potential distractions, concentrate on what you do. You may need to:

- Sit and work in a quiet area, away from every one's eyes.
- Hand your pager to a colleague for cover.
- Take the phone off the socket, turn off your electronic tablet.
- Close the door, put a "do not disturb" sign on the door, lock the door.

Minimise time looking up information

Have easily accessible information that you regularly need in your day to day practise, rather than having to keep looking for it every time the need arises. Having regularly needed information at your fingertips, can save you valuable time.

You may:

- Carry a pocket size-reference clinical book, relevant to your current post. A book that you can refer to easily and one likely to give you the necessary answers. Alternatively, have access to a relevant electronic clinical book, website or app on your phone or tablet.
- Make your own lists of tests to order, or investigations to request, for commonly encountered clinical conditions. You may have a list of tests to order for acute onset epigastric pain, acute onset hip pain, pyrexia of unknown origin, recent onset weight loss. Avoid relying on memory and hence leaving out some of these tests.
- Have a list of commonly used phone numbers or pagers, rather than having to look them up each time. You may need to ring up the pathology lab to order urgent blood tests, or ask for an urgent lumbar puncture gram stain. You may have to ring from the ward, from the Emergency Department, from the hospital corridor, but the switchboard may not be answering.
- Have a list of clinical diagnostic codes or surgical procedure codes. You may have to provide clinical codes when admitting a patient, when listing a patient for surgery or after carrying a surgical procedure. Such codes may aid remuneration of yourself or your institution, for the work provided. Rather than having to go through endless lists of codes each time, keep the ones you most commonly use, in an easily accessible format.
- Have a list of equipment you need for commonly performed procedures, surgical or otherwise. You may be asked to perform such procedures in the middle of the night, in a ward you attend for the first time, with staff you never met before. You may have a list of what you need to catheterise a patient; what type of catheter, what size, local anaesthetic agent, or volume of fluid to inflate the catheter balloon.

Avoid Procrastination

Procrastination is like a credit card: it's a lot of fun until you get the bill

Christopher Parker [1]

Procrastination describes the habit of putting off things or unnecessarily delaying tasks that should be promptly completed [3]. Avoid postponing for tomorrow, what should and can be done today. You may keep putting off the work-based assessments, the surgical logbook update, the medico legal reports, completing the discharge summaries or the disability assessment forms, copying the drug charts, responding to a complaint, replying to an email, going through those patients' records for the upcoming audit meeting, writing or submitting that research article, getting the presentation slides ready.

Putting off things results in workload mounting, results in unnecessary worry and anxiety. If postponing becomes a habit, try and break it. In doing so, you may consider the reasons for avoiding those tasks, to help find suitable solutions:

- Tasks not interesting- appreciate that not all tasks will be as stimulating or exciting. Some will be boring or daunting, but still have to be completed. Rather than concentrating on how uninspired you will be whilst doing those tasks, try and see how relieved you may feel once they are out of the way.
- Tasks not rewarding or of minimal training value– service provision and training go hand and hand. Something new can be learnt even from the most repetitive task.
- Tasks not important– all tasks have a relative value, work out what that is. Completing discharge summaries promptly may ensure patients are discharged on time, allowing new ones to move from Emergency Department trolleys to ward beds.
- Not sure where to start- break the task down into small segments, small fragments that can easily be tackled.
- Not skilled or trained- get training, ask for guidance.
- Something else keeps turning up- put such tasks high up on your to-do list and get them done early. Try and complete tasks as soon as you come across them, rather than putting them on the side for later on.

Allow for the Unexpected

What we anticipate seldom occurs: but what we least expect generally happens
Benjamin Disraeli [1]

Anticipate that some tasks will take longer than planned, answers may take longer to receive, solutions may take longer to figure out. Do not leave completion of tasks and meeting of deadlines, for the last moment. Avoid working on the edge and assuming all will go smoothly, according to plan, all will fall in place on time. Allow for the unexpected:

- A patient may crash, disrupting your routine ward round.
- The appendix may be too inflamed and stuck, taking time to mobilise and remove, prolonging your operating list.
- A patient may present with a long list of questions to your clinic, which take time to answer.
- Your trainer may be on holidays or have a full schedule, and not be available to sign you off in time for your upcoming training program assessment.
- Some audit records may be off site and take longer to get, for that next audit presentation.
- You may be kept up all night whilst on call, too tired to finish the research abstract that needs submitting.
- Your clinical post may be busier than expected, with less free time to study for the upcoming exams.
- The medical illustration department may be overwhelmed with lots of last minute requests for posters printing, with yours having to be pushed down the queue.
- The article you need for the upcoming departmental teaching may not be available locally, and has to be obtained through an inter-library loan.
- Your laptop may crash, just as you are about to submit the next post application.

Try and be one step ahead. Avoid working on a tight schedule. Allow time for late starts, interruptions, emergencies, overruns. Allow for you not being able to work at full speed, allow for others not being able to perform at their best.

You may be assigned a new task, you may be asked to take on a new project. You may be asked to write a research proposal, carry out an audit, write an article, prepare a presentation, organise the departmental teaching, device a new protocol, revise a care pathway, organise next year's rota. Set realistic deadlines. Be an optimist but also a pragmatist before you make promises. Err towards caution. It may be better to under-promise and over-perform, rather than overpromise and under-deliver. It is better to impress with a prompt delivery, rather than disappoint with a failed promise of a prompt deadline.

In estimating how much time you may need for a task, and what deadlines to set up you may consider:

- What other work do you already have scheduled and how much time is that likely to take? How much free time does that leave you for the new task? Could you drop other tasks to concentrate on the new one?
- Is it likely that new additional work could turn up during the time under consideration? If additional work keeps turning up now, it is highly likely it will do so in the future. Is a busy or quiet time of the year coming up?
- Break the task into small components, as it may be easier to grasp their size, and hence estimate the time that each of those may take.
- Does completion of the task depend solely on you or do you rely on input from others? If relying on others, how much time will they take? Are others reliable and available to deliver on time? How much influence do you have as to when they deliver?
- If the task does prove to take longer than expected, can you call upon additional staff, help and resources, to make up for lost time?
- What happened last time you undertook a similar task? What delays occurred then? What lessons were learnt?

Work out how much time you think you will need. Then add some more, and even some more again.

Have to-Do Lists

The project may be the lion, but the list is your whip

Adam Savage [1]

Prepare lists of tasks to do. Such lists may be hand written or in electronic format. You may carry to-do lists on paper sheets, notebooks, or electronic tablets. Use whichever format suits you, whatever format enables you to quickly add new tasks, and cross off those completed. Some situations where to-do lists may be useful:

- You are on out-of hours duty, you get calls for referrals from the Emergency Department, wards, community doctors; make a record of each of these and get the contact of the referrer, in case you need more information.
- You do a ward round; make a list of investigations you need to request for each patient, to be acted upon.
- You are doing a research project; make a list of experiments to do, collaborators to meet, articles to read.
- You are revising for your post-graduate exams; make a list of topics you need to cover, clinical signs you need to see, clinical diagnoses to make, courses to attend.
- You want to further develop your surgical skills; make a list of operations you want to observe, to assist in or perform.

Lists help you easily see what is outstanding, allow you to prioritise the various tasks, and help you avoid relying on memory. Lists may even give you the satisfaction every time a completed task is crossed off. When it comes to drawing up lists you may consider:

- For each item make an adequate meaningful record, easy to action when its turn comes.
- Make a record as to when each item was added, as that may guide as to when to act upon.
- Mark the tasks as high and low priority. Keep re-assessing the list, and re-prioritise as needed.
- Break down tasks into smaller components that make it easier to see what is outstanding.
- Distinguish the tasks that only you can do from those that can be delegated.

Prioritise

The key is not to prioritise what's on your schedule, but to schedule your priorities
Stephen Covey [1]

Allocate priority to various tasks. We often think of triage in the war field or in triaging patients in the Emergency Department. However, triaging is a vital skill for a doctor's day to day professional life. Time is limited, so many tasks to be completed. Some tasks must be done promptly, others can wait. Identify those tasks that matter the most and ensure they are done first. Prioritising is a skill that needs to be mastered.

You may prioritise according to clinical urgency and importance, according to up-coming deadlines, according to waiting time, according to availability of skills and resources. Consider:

- You may prioritise the assessment of a ward chesty patient with dropping blood pressure, as compared to reviewing stable long stayers whose condition has not changed.
- You may prioritise rushing to surgery a nasty fracture with a pulseless arm, as compared to plastering an ankle sprain.
- You may prioritise ringing the radiologist to request a brain scan in newly-onset blurred speech, as compared to ordering routine post-knee replacement radiographs.
- You may prioritise the completion of discharge summaries for patients to be discharged early in the day (to free beds and admit others), as compared to putting out routine blood test requests.
- You may prioritise the write up of an abstract for a scientific meeting with a looming deadline, as compared to writing up the detailed methodology for a newly thought project.
- You may prioritise reviewing a case for which you are likely to need senior input, before your boss sets off for an off-site clinic.
- You may be handed a list of patients waiting to be seen at the start of your on-call duty. Who is to be seen first?

Obtain the necessary information from other healthcare staff or patients themselves, to enable you to quickly prioritise various tasks. Know as to who is the best source of such information. You may consider:

- You may be looking after lots of patients in the ward, and you are ready to start your morning ward round. Ask the night shift nursing staff, or the night shift ward doctor, as to how patients have been overnight, to identify problems that need prompt attention.
- You may be on call and turn up to the Emergency Department with many referrals to be seen. Scan the referrals and prioritise the order of review, firstly according to clinical urgency and then wait time. Ask the charge nurse if anything has changed in patients' condition since their referral, rather than simply relying on the referral charts.

- You may be handed over by a colleague a list of jobs to do or patients to see. Ask that colleague if there are any patients that need immediate attention, or any tasks that should be done first.

In deciding how to prioritise, clinical importance and urgency come first. Make a list of outstanding jobs to put a structure into what is waiting, and mark on the list the clinical priority of each. If you could do only one job, which one would that be? With more and more doctors working shifts, outstanding jobs have to be passed from one shift to the other. You may be worried of the perception you give, if you pass on tasks which have been waiting a long time. Others may wonder how you could not have done those jobs earlier on in the day. If, however, clinical need dictates that you deal with other tasks first, then do so. The performance of institutions and departments is increasingly assessed using targets of length of patients' wait; wait in the Emergency Department, wait to be seen in clinic, wait to surgery [4–6]. You may occasionally feel pressure to deal with long waiters first, pressures of the consequences if targets are not met. Again, clinical urgency takes priority. Apologise to those waiting long, and explain why you did not attend to them earlier. Most may well agree that the sicker should be dealt first. Prioritise, deal with the most unwell first.

Delegate

I either delegate something, I dump it, or I deal with it

Daniel Doctoroff [1]

We can not do absolutely everything, complete all tasks in person. No matter how talented we are, how enthusiastic, committed, keen, skilled and hard working we feel, we often have to ask others for help, we often have to delegate some tasks to others. These may be clinical, administrative, technical, managerial or other tasks. For tasks which can be done by others, ask them to do so. It is not a sign of weakness or failure but a skill that combines the ability to organise, prioritise, and work effectively as part of a team. It is a skill that requires the ability to recognise which tasks can be delegated and to whom they can be delegated, in order to ensure their prompt, safe and successful completion.

You may ask a colleague to clinically assess a patient in clinic or the ward, take bloods, order blood tests, speak to a radiologist for an investigation, suture the surgical incision wound, collect data for an upcoming audit, counsel a patient about a research trial. You may ask the scrub nurse to prep the patient whilst you are scrubbing, your secretary to set up the projector ready for your presentation, the rota master to print the rota guidelines for the induction of the new trainees. You may ask your juniors or peers to lead the medical students' teaching, represent you in a multi-disciplinary meeting, or liaise with a specialist team to ensure prompt assessment of an unwell patient.

Share the jobs rather than piling them up. It may initially be faster and easier to do everything yourself rather than showing others how to do things. You may be able to do things much better than everyone else. However, if you delegate, whilst offering guidance as needed, others may develop the knowledge and skills, to carry those tasks under minimal supervision, an important component of professional development and training. Delegate important tasks rather than simply those you do not fancy doing. As others become more confident in sharing your work, and as you develop the confidence they will deliver, give them tasks which need more responsibility. Show that you value their contribution, that you trust them to follow things through. Sharing may help you all work towards a common goal.

Give Others the Time They Need

If they try to rush me, I always say, I've only got one other speed and it's slower
Glenn Ford [1]

You may feel like the centre of the world, you may enjoy having what you ask for without delays, your deadlines may be the most important, your tasks the most critical.

However, the people we work with have their own tasks, their own deadlines to meet, so many others to please. They may really want to help you out but other jobs are holding them back. They may want to do their best, but cannot just drop all they are doing. Hence, give them ample time to meet your requests. You may consider:

- Give your trainers ample time for setting up your final sign off meeting, in time for your training program paperwork submission deadline.
- Give ample time to the medical records department to pull out the notes, in time for the next audit meeting presentation.
- Give your co-researchers ample time to comment on your research funding proposal, in time for the application deadline.
- Give ample warning to your clinic administrators for your holidays, to re-arrange clinic appointments.
- Give ample time to your secretary to type your response to a patient's complaint, in time for the response deadline.
- Give ample time to the ward staff to bring a patient down to clinic for plaster change. Let them know from the start of the clinic, if not from the day before.
- Give the library sufficient time to get those references for your research introduction, rather than waiting until the end when you are about to start writing up your thesis.
- Give the journal sufficient time to consider your article submission, for that long awaited decision to boost your curriculum vitae (CV).

Show that you are organised, you respect and value the time of others, that you can plan ahead.

Have a Routine, Follow a System

We are what we repeatedly do. Excellence, then, is not an act, but a habit

Aristotle [1]

Some of your activities may be scheduled or structured by others, but some will be directly guided by you. Develop a routine or system as to how you do things. It may be a routine with regards timing, methodology, approach. You may consider:

- If covering multiple wards, have set times when you go round. If staff know that you will come round, they will be more likely to leave non-urgent jobs till then, rather than keep paging you. Tell staff when you will be back. As many tasks can wait, ask staff to make a list, and explain that you will do regular ward rounds. Otherwise, you may end up rushing from ward to ward to do tasks as they arise.
- If you do a weekly ward round, have fixed time and starting place and stick to it. Staff will wait for you, will do their best to ensure someone is available to join you, rather than turning up and looking for staff to go round.
- If you have a time when you will go through your non urgent administration work, your secretary will keep it for then rather than ringing every time something new turns up.
- If you are a doing a certain procedure or operation the same way, same sequence, and using the same instruments and equipment every time, then staff will know what to get ready for you, and will be able to follow your operating. You may even be handed the next instrument before you ask for it!
- If you are discharging patients have a system as to what thrombo-prophylaxis you prescribe, when you follow up patients in clinic, how you communicate with out of hospital carers.

If you keep changing your habits, you may have to explain this from scratch every time to all those working with you. If you keep changing you may confuse everyone. Stick to a system. It allows others to get used to your ways. It would be unfair to expect others to lay the red carpet if you keep changing your habits for no reason. Practise makes better. If you stick to a system you can get better and faster at what you do. There will be exceptions, but that is understandable.

Leading a Ward Round

Organizing is what you do before you do something, so that when you do it, it is not all mixed up

Alan Alexander Milne [1]

As a doctor you may have to lead a ward round. Often it is a junior member of the team that takes the seniors round, informing them about any new patients admitted after an on-call duty, or informing them about existing patients, about their current state, the decisions made and the decisions that need to be made. Being able to lead an efficient ward round during your day to day work or on call cover is an important skill to develop. It incorporates many of the organisational skills that this chapter addresses, and allows you to put many of them into practise [7–12].

A ward round aims to review patients' clinical condition, make, adjust, or change the underlying diagnosis, assess progress, review investigation and treatment plans, formulate discharge arrangements. A ward round gives the opportunity to check investigation results, drug charts, fluid and dietary prescriptions, outputs, thromboprophylaxis, mobilisation status, surgical wounds. A ward round may ensure that clear communication about patients' care is established amongst healthcare workers. A ward round may allow communication with patients and relatives regarding condition, progress and future plans.

Aim to lead a well paced, structured ward round, rather than thinking what to do next, where to go, wandering purpose-less around. The following may help you achieve that:

- Know where and when the ward round takes place, and be there on time.
- Remind any healthcare staff that will join you (nurses, physiotherapists, occupational therapists, pharmacists) of the upcoming ward round.
- Know where your patients are, as patients get moved around the hospital to different wards and within a ward to different bays. Walking all the way to the Emergency Department at the other end of the hospital, just to find out the patient has been moved to a ward, is not an effective way of time utilisation. Consider ringing outlier wards to ensure patients are still there, before you set off.
- Plan as how you will go round, plan the order of seeing patients. Prioritise according to clinical urgency, and then according to other factors such as patient's location. If a patient is very unwell and their senior review happens to coincide with the ward round, start from that case.
- Have at hand a summary of the condition of each patient, including the timing of important milestones (date of admission, days from significant event, days post surgery or other procedure, days post commencement of new treatment). Have information with regards to discharge arrangements, as such arrangements may have to be initiated early.
- Have at hand up to date investigations and test results. Electronic tablets may make that easy [11].
- Have checklists to ensure all relevant issues are covered.

- If the ward round involves looking at radiographs, get those out, leave them by the bedside, or ensure they are easily accessible. If radiographs are in electronic form, ensure you can easily get to see them.
- Ensure medical records and other charts are available, and know where they are. The records of patients awaiting surgery may be kept in a separate part of the ward compared to those of the remaining patients. The medication charts may have been sent to the hospital pharmacy to order new drugs.
- Ensure any equipment you may need is available. You may need a doppler to look for pulses, an ophthalmoscope for fundoscopy, are these available?
- Have the details of your patients ready. Double check your list, make sure that all patients to be seen are indeed on your list, and that all patients on the list are indeed to be seen.
- Know the current state of patients. If you admitted a patient the previous night, whilst on call, visit the patient in the morning prior to the ward round, to determine how they have been overnight. Are they better, have they deteriorated? Have they been seen by the other team from whom you asked an assessment?
- Know any specific requests made or questions raised by your seniors in their last ward round, and have the answers to those ready. Know the plan of action of the last ward round. This might have been a request for a further opinion, investigation or assessment.
- Make notes in the patients' records as you go along, or make separate notes and come and write back in the patients' records at the end of the ward round. Even if your seniors are dictating a typed letter, as a means of documenting their ward round findings, still write in the notes, as typed letters may take time to reach the charts.
- Carry investigation forms or other referral forms, as some of these may need to be completed and signed by seniors.

References

1. Famous quotes at BrainyQuote. www.brainyquote.com. Accessed on 23 Sept 2014.
2. Batejat D, Lagarde D, Navelet Y, Binder M. Evaluation of the attention span of 10,000 school children 8–11 years of age. Arch Pediatr. 1999;6(4):406–15.
3. Oxford dictionaries. www.oxforddictionaries.com. Accessed on 23 Sept 2014.
4. Dimakou S, Parkin D, Devlin N, Appleby J. Identifying the impact of government targets on waiting times in the NHS. Health Care Manag Sci. 2009;12(1):1–10.
5. Appleby J, Boyle S, Devlin N, Harley M, Harrison A, Thorlby R. Do English NHS waiting time targets distort treatment priorities in orthopaedic surgery? J Health Serv Res Policy. 2005;10(3):167–72.
6. Vezyridis P, Timmons S. National targets, process transformation and local consequences in an NHS emergency department (ED): a qualitative study. BMC Emerg Med. 2014;14:12.
7. Royal College of Physicians, Royal College of Nursing. Ward rounds in medicine: principles for best practice. London: RCP; 2012.
8. Herring R, Desai T, Caldwell G. Quality and safety at the point of care: how long should a ward round take? Clin Med. 2011;11(1):20–2.
9. Cohn A. The ward round: what it is and what it can be. Br J Hosp Med (Lond). 2014;75(6):C82–5.
10. Sharma S, Peters MJ, PICU/NICU Risk Action Group. Safety by DEFAULT': introduction and impact of a paediatric ward round checklist. Crit Care. 2013;17(5):R232.
11. Baysari MT, Adams K, Lehnbom EC, Westbrook JI, Day RO. iPad use at the bedside: a tool for engaging patients in care processes during ward-rounds? Int Med J. 2014;44:986–90. doi:10.1111/imj.12518.
12. Krautter M, Koehl-Hackert N, Nagelmann L, Jünger J, Norcini J, Tekian A, Nikendei C. Improving ward round skills. Med Teach. 2014;36(9):783–8.

Chapter 3
Communication

Communication is the passing and receiving information with verbal, written, or other means. Communication also refers to the development of relations with those we interact. Effective communication refers to the exchange of accurate and correct information, but also refers to an appropriate manner with which such information is transmitted.

Communication skills are vital both in dealing with patients, their friends and relatives, but also other healthcare workers. Whatever the form of communication selected, it is important to ensure that the desired message is delivered and clearly understood by the receiver.

This chapter initially addresses certain basic skills of communication, with a particular reference to relational communication. The need of maintaining confidentiality is emphasised and particular areas of verbal, written, and electronic communication are addressed. Systems that can allow structured communication are presented, and the role of effective communication in promoting safe clinical practise is discussed. Advice is given regarding special situations of communication including breaking bad news, consenting, and writing a business case.

© Springer International Publishing Switzerland 2015
C. Panayiotou Charalambous, *Career Skills for Doctors*,
DOI 10.1007/978-3-319-13479-6_3

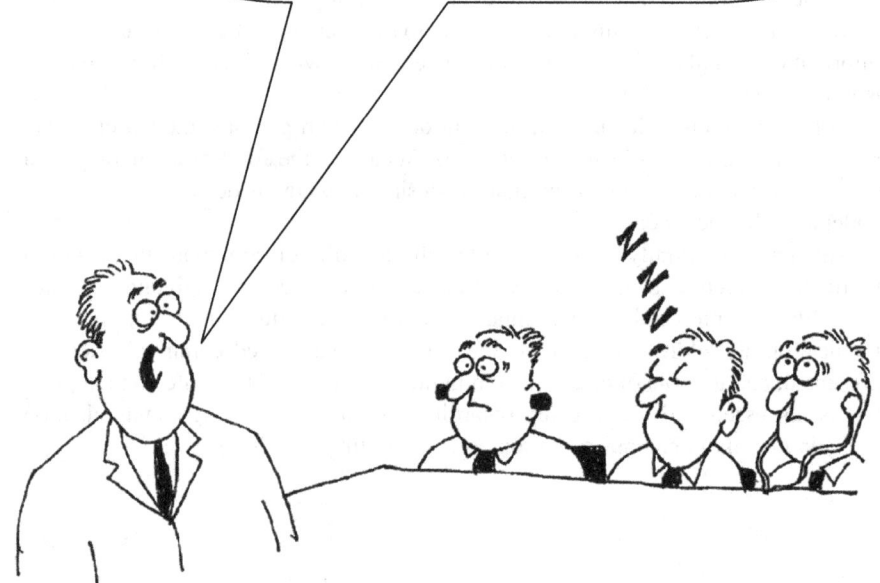

Communication: The Basics

It is not the voice that commands the story; it is the ear

Italo Calvino [1]

Whatever the means of communication you use, the basic principles remain the same. Be polite, respectful, courteous, friendly, and approachable in dealing both with patients and other staff. In a 2008 article in the New England Journal of Medicine, Michael Khan, a Boston psychiatrist, introduced the term "Etiquette based medicine" to introduce the use of "good manners", in the patient-doctor interaction [2]. Khan believed that patients may give particular importance to whether doctors are respectful and attentive. He recommended that for a patient to have a satisfying experience, doctors should, in their first meeting with a hospital patient:

1. Ask permission to enter the patient's room, and wait for answer.
2. Show their identity badge and introduce themselves.
3. Shake hands.
4. Sit down and smile if appropriate.
5. Explain their role in the medical team.
6. Ask as to how the patient feels for being in hospital.

Khan's recommendations could be applied not only to dealing with patients, but also in dealing with colleagues and other staff. In direct personal contact consider the following:

• Get to know people's names and address them with that. In a busy environment, with staff having different working patterns, you may often see new faces. You may not have met the nurse assisting you in clinic before, the radiographer screening your patients in theatre, the junior doctor covering the wards, the secretary typing your clinic letters. Ask who they are and get to know them. They will appreciate that you took the time and effort to find out their name and use it as such. You may not be keen at speaking to strangers in the street, why should you be doing so at work?
• Introduce yourself rather than assuming the other person knows who you are. They may not be able to read your badge, may be new starters, may not have heard of you before.
• Give your title and explain your role. You may be wearing your suit, a white coat, your scrubs, having a stethoscope round your neck. Still explain who you are and why you are there.
• Introduce your team and explain their role. You may be in charge, the one making decisions, the rest may be taking orders or be shadowing you to learn. If you are leading the encounter introduce all those present. Acknowledge the presence and contribution of all those around you, to avoid others wondering as to who all these strangers surrounding you are.
• Look at people when you address them or speak to them. Avoid staring at a radiograph whilst asking questions to someone standing behind you, avoid making computer entries whilst taking a clinical history, avoid checking your

emails whilst a junior is seeking your attention. Pause and address the person you are speaking to. Give them the moment they deserve.

- Use plain language, easily understood by the person you are referring to. Avoid complex, technical terms, no matter how sophisticated they may sound.
- Minimise interruptions. Close the door, draw the curtain, concentrate on the person you are communicating with.

Albert Mehrabian, Professor Emeritus of Psychology, at the University of California, Los Angeles, USA, in his work on human communication, stresses that there are three elements of face to face communication: words, tone of voice, and non-verbal behaviours (such as facial expression) [3–5]. Mehrabian proposes that when an individual talks about their likes or dislikes, 7 % of communication is achieved by words, 38 % by tone of voice and 55 % by body language.

- Use the appropriate body language. If you walk in a room looking stung up, is it really the best approach to motivate and attract the support of others? If you deliver a lecture standing rigidly still, will you infuse the audience with passion? If you attend a meeting and sit leaning back looking at the ceiling, are you truly engaging?
- Use the appropriate tone, the correct volume, and right pace. You may be a soft talker, but may need to raise your voice for others to pay attention. You may be a fast talker, but may need to slow down if others have difficulty following you, especially if they just met you.
- Use appropriate terms when addressing others. Address your patients, colleagues and seniors with their title and surname, unless they specifically ask you to refer to them otherwise. It may be unwise to start calling your professor "Bill", just because you overheard the senior ward sister addressing him by his first name. It may be unwise to start calling your senior "mate" or "man", no matter how friendly and approachable they seem, no matter how widely such expressions are used. Even if you are on first names, should you not be referring to your senior with their full name and title when talking to others? However, if asked by a senior to address them with their first name, try and do so; respect and courtesy can still be practised, even for those who are on first name terms.
- The world is a tiny neighbourhood. Doctors may move to practise in lands away from their country of origin, patients may live or work away from home. Having good grasp of the language of the place you are practising in, is essential to ensure proper communication. If your accent or your patient's accent hinders communication, ask someone local to help you communicate. If doing a ward round and the patient has poor hearing or cannot appreciate your accent, ask the patient's nurse or other carer for help. A nurse, who spends more time with a patient, may have found a way round. If you and the patient can not speak the same language use a translator, preferably someone unrelated to the patient, rather than just assuming information will get across.
- Listen; communication is a two way process. It is not just about passing information but also about receiving. Try and be a keen listener rather than just doing the talking. You are more likely to learn something new by hearing someone else

speak, rather than if you do all the talking. Listen to what others have to say, give them time and attention. Listen to silence. You may be chairing a meeting and after your preaching talk no one else speaks. You may give a talk and no one questions you at the end. Sometimes silence speaks louder than protests and screams.

- Use open ended rather than close ended questions, to allow others to open themselves, and tell you about their opinions or troubles. You may obtain more information if you use open ended questions rather than asking for specifics. People may concentrate on what they value most, on what they feel is important, if given an open forum. Direct questions may provide specific facts, but may fail to give the whole picture. Consider getting the bigger picture first prior to concentrating on details.

Relational Communication

My belief is that communication is the best way to create strong relationships
Jada Pinkett Smith [1]

Communication refers to the exchange of correct and accurate information, but also to the formation of healthy interpersonal relationships both with patients and other staff.

Relational communication is described by Guerrero, Andersen and Afifi, in their book "Close Encounters: Communication in Relationships", as a subset of inter-personal communication that focuses on messages exchanged within relationships [6]. They go on to say that "relational communication reflects the nature of a relationship at a particular time. Communication constitutes and defines relationships. In other words communication is the substance of close relationships". Five principles of relational communication [6] are:

1. Relationships are the result of repeated interactions, which are partly communication interactions.
2. Messages may have different meanings in various relationships. Hence the message must be interpreted within a context or relationship.
3. Communication reflects the nature of relationships. Relational messages have been classified into seven types [7]: dominance/submission, level of intimacy (affection, trust, inclusion), degree of similarity, task-social interactions, formality/informality, degree of social composure, emotional arousal or activation.
4. Relational communication, like relationships themselves, is dynamic.
5. Relational communication may follow linear (constant progress or deterioration) or non-linear (ups and downs) patterns.

Step et al. [8] suggest that "relational communication contributes to a climate for interaction that can facilitate or inhibit effective communication outcomes".

Using the study tool shown in Table 3.1, Shay et al. [9], looked at the factors associated with patients evaluating a physician's relational communication as positive. They reported that simple physician acts, like asking more unprompted questions, and encouraging expression of concerns, led to more positive rating of the interaction. Interestingly, neither the time spent with the patient nor the time the patient had to spend in the waiting room prior to getting seen, were associated with how relational communication was rated.

Orioles et al. [10] asked the parents of patients hospitalized in a pediatric intensive care unit and bone marrow transplant unit, how they perceived their physicians' inter-personal behaviors. They identified 11 inter-personal behaviors considered as important by parents. These included empathy, availability, treating the child as an individual, respecting the parents' knowledge of the child, allowing hope, correct body language, thoroughness, exceeding duty requirements, accountability, willingness to be questioned, and attention to the child's suffering.

Table 3.1 Items used by Shay et al. [9] to assess how patients evaluated relational communication by their physicians

Relational communication scale items used in the factor score
1. My doctor was interested in talking to me
2. My doctor seemed to care if I liked him/her
3. My doctor was sincere
4. My doctor wanted me to trust him/her
5. My doctor was willing to listen to me
6. My doctor was open to my ideas
7. My doctor was honest in communicating with me
8. My doctor seemed nervous in my presence
9. My doctor was comfortable interacting with me
10. My doctor wanted to cooperate with me

Patients rated the above items during their post-visit survey on a seven-point Likert scale ranging from (1) strongly disagree to (7) strongly agree
Reprinted with permission

Confidentiality

Confidentiality is a virtue of the loyal, as loyalty is the virtue of faithfulness
Edwin Louis Cole [1]

Take all steps to ensure that confidentiality is respected and not violated. This applies to both dealing with patients but also other staff. Use common sense, and take all possible steps to minimise breaching of confidentiality. Follow the data protection rules of your organisation, the guidance of your regulatory body, follow the rules of the land. You may consider:

- Should you be dictating loudly a letter about a patient in the corridor or in the coffee room, in front of colleagues or non-medical staff?
- If your favourite clinic receptionist asked you what was wrong with her neighbour, who you saw in clinic that morning, should you be telling?
- Should you be telling your partner about the medical condition of a prominent village figure?
- Should you be stopping at a patient's house for a home visit on your way to taking your partner shopping?
- Should you be keeping in your portfolio a copy of your logbook with identifiable patient's details?
- Should you be including in your national audit lecture a radiograph with the patient's details at the top?
- Should you be keeping information about patients on non-encrypted, non-password protected memory stick or laptop? What if it gets lost?
- Should you be taking written medical records home? What if you left your bag in the train?
- Should you be passing information to a patient's employer without the patient's consent?
- Should you be emailing identifiable information about a patient without using appropriate encryption? What if the email goes astray or your email account gets hacked?
- Should you be leaving, at the end of the consultation, a computer on with a patient's radiographs and details exposed, whilst you move next door to see someone else? What if another patient walks in?
- If dealing with a patient involved in criminal activity, or if there is concern about a communicable disease, how can you balance acting in the public interest with the need to respect an individual's confidentiality?

Confidentiality is at the centre of patient-doctor relationships. Consider the implications if confidentiality were to be compromised, both to patient and you alike.

The same rules apply in dealing with confidential issues of colleagues and other staff. Others may confide to you their personal circumstances, the challenges they are going through, ask you for a listening ear, for direction and advice. You may be made aware of confidential information because of your position, your seniority or role. You may overhear a telephone conversation or coffee room talk. You may consider:

- Should you be telling other staff the medical reasons for one of your juniors being off sick?
- Should you be telling about the family troubles a colleague is going through?
- Should you be telling how poor the performance of one of your juniors was in an interview that you recently chaired?
- Should you be telling others about your colleague facing disciplinary action?
- You may have reviewed a research article submitted to a journal but is still not published. Should you be telling your research fellows about its weaknesses?
- You may have reviewed a research grant application proposal the decision for which is still awaited. Should you be telling other researches about it?
- A colleague may be applying for a new post but does not wish people at work to know until it is secured. Should you be telling others about the reference the colleague asked you to provide?

If you have been entrusted with confidential information, keep that trust. If others asked you to keep their troubles to yourself, then do so. It helps you build good reputation and gain respect in the workplace. If others know that what they tell you will be like front page news, then it is unlikely they will confide to you again.

Summarising and Systematically Presenting

The most valuable of all talents is that of never using two words when one will do
Thomas Jefferson [1]

In the medical school we are often taught to take a thorough clinical history and carry a full clinical examination, the recording of which may be pages and pages long. We may then be rewarded for presenting the whole story to our tutors, for giving all positive and negative facts. We may be praised for not leaving anything out, for covering all aspects and angles of the story.

In contrast, as a practising doctor, you are often required to collect this information but present it in a succinct, summarised form. Time is limited, everyone is rushed, decisions must be made, actions must be taken. You may be presenting the patients admitted during a busy on call, you may be leading a busy ward round, you may be assessing and presenting patients in the out-patients clinic, you may be presenting patients turning up for surgery, you may be handing over a list of cases to be seen during the night shift, you may be referring to another team for specialised opinion, you may be ringing up for senior advice, you may be writing a hospital discharge summary.

Try to develop the skill of picking out and presenting all vital information, but putting aside anything which is less relevant or less important. It is a skill not to present everything but to present what is essential, and related to the message you are trying to convey. It is a skill not to give a long essay but a succinct summary, one that can be easily grasped in a busy clinical environment.

Have a system as how you communicate such information which may be applied in verbal or written form, which may be employed in multiple clinical settings and contexts. The SBAR (situation, background, assessment, recommendation) [11] and SOAP (subjective, objective, assessment, plan) [12] communication schemes may help you present information in a structured way. SBAR was initially designed for nurses briefing physicians in an obstetrics unit [11], whereas SOAP was used as guidance of recording in medical charts [12]. Both incorporate the reporting of information gathered from the patient, carers, or other witnesses, and clinical findings gathered by the clinician. These are combined to develop your overall impression or opinion, and finally formulate a further management plan.

These communication schemes are summarised below:

S-ituation – what is happening
B-ackground – previous relevant history
A-ssessment – clinical findings
R-ecomendation – what needs to happen, further plan

S-ubjective – clinical symptoms and previous history
O-bjective – clinical signs
A-ssessment – clinician's impressions
P-lan – action needed

An example would be:

<u>Situation</u>:	52 year old male, just presented to Emergency Department with acute onset chest pain and nausea
<u>**B**ackground</u>:	Clumsy, tachycardic, no history of heart disease, but heavy smoker
<u>**A**ssessment</u>:	ECG shows ST elevation
<u>**R**ecommend</u>:	To have urgent angioplasty

<u>**S**ubjective</u>:	52 year old male, acute onset chest pain, nausea, no previous heart disease, heavy smoker
<u>**O**bjective</u>:	Clumsy, tachycardic
<u>**A**ssessment</u>:	ECG shows ST elevation
<u>**P**lan</u>:	To have urgent angioplasty

The development of succinct and systematic presentation skills may take time. Keep practising to get better.

Communication and Safety

The single biggest problem with communication is the illusion that it has taken place
George Bernand Shaw [1]

Doing no harm is paramount in health care. Yet, when things go wrong or do not go according to plan, failure of communication is cited as one of the main causes. The Joint Commission for Hospital Accreditation in the USA, identified communication failures as one of the root causes in more than 60 % of 7,194 sentinel events from 2004 to 2013. Such events included operating on the wrong patient or wrong site, carrying out the wrong procedure, unintended retention of foreign objects (such as swabs) at surgery, radiation overdose, medication errors, and delay in treatment [13]. Several aspects of communication may help improve safety, and these are described below.

Use Similar Language

This refers to using structured communication systems or clinical management pathways, so that all participants are aware of what the messages mean. The ALS (Advanced Life Support) and ATLS (Advanced Trauma Life Support) systems, commonly used in clinical practise, put structure in how to resuscitate a collapsed patient or approach a trauma patient [14, 15]. Clinicians trained in these systems are thus able to "speak the same language" when undertaking such crucial tasks. Avoid abbreviations or technical terms that may not be easily understood by others.

Ensure the Message Has Been Received

Ask the receiver to repeat the message to confirm their understanding. Even though one speaks and one hears, the message may still be lost.

Brief/Debrief

Brief and debrief prior to and after major events. Briefings ensure that all participants have a shared understanding of what is about to happen, any risks involved, and any alternative plans. The World Health Organisation Surgical Safety Checklist provides a structured briefing prior to commencing surgery. It also allows debriefing at the end of surgery to highlight what was done, any problems encountered and which could be avoided next time, as well as further actions necessary [16, 17].

Alerting Systems for When Things Are Not Right

In 1978 a United Airlines plane crashed near the Portland International airport in Oregon, USA. The landing gear of the plane failed and the crew became so absorbed with addressing the failed gear, overlooking that fuel was running out. The plane crashed due to fuel exhaustion. Cockpit recordings suggested that one of the crash causes was the failure of the first officer and the flight engineer to successfully communicate their concerns about the plane's fuel state to the captain [18]. This, and other similar events, led to the introduction of cockpit resource management, a system of providing training as how to act in situations where error can have dramatic consequences. Since then, parallels have been drawn between cockpit resource management and communication in healthcare [19–22].

You may find yourself in a situation where you feel that things are not right. Someone maybe about to administer a treatment that may not be appropriate, someone maybe overlooking a critical clinical sign, and you need to communicate effectively your concerns. The person you are trying to communicate with may be higher up in hierarchy, which may complicate matters even further.

Several communication systems have been described for such situations, to help you make your concerns explicit. Three such systems are CUS (Concerned, Uncertain, Safety) [23], the Two-Challenge rule [24], and the Assertive Statement [25]. These put a structure in how to escalate concerns and attract attention to those.

The CUS technique was developed by the Agency for Healthcare Research and Quality in the USA [23]. This is described below:

C-oncern	"I am <u>concerned</u> we should not be doing this"
U-nsure	"I am <u>uncertain</u> that we can do this"
S-afety	"I feel it is <u>unsafe</u> to do this"
	"We should <u>stop</u> and not do this"

The Two-Challenge rule, is an alternative approach, originating from the aviation industry, and recommended in the Institute of Medicine's 1999 report "To err is human" [26]. If a pilot is challenged twice and does not respond appropriately, then the assistance takes control. Even though this approach may not directly apply to healthcare, it gives a guide that if after two challenges an appropriate response is not achieved then going up the chain of command is needed.

The Assertive Statement was originally developed by Dr Jerry Berlin while developing Crew Resource Management courses for the airlines in the late 1980s. It is used by Jay Hopkins of the Error Prevention Institute in Preventing Human Error seminars [25] and involves:

- Get the person's attention: "Dr Jones"
- State your concern: "I am very concerned that we are giving the wrong dose of heparin"
- State the problem as you see it: "The heparin dose is too high for the patient's weight"

- Propose a solution: "We should stop and re-calculate the dose"
- Obtain agreement (or buy-in): "Do you agree, doctor?"

If you are on the receiving end and someone is questioning your decision then stop, listen and reconsider. Do not just brush it off. Enquire why is the challenger saying that? Could you be doing something wrong? Respect the challenger no matter how junior they are, whether a doctor or not.

Handover

Handover is defined as "the transfer of professional responsibility and accountability for some or all aspects of care for a patient, or group of patients to another person or professional group on a temporary or permanent basis" [27].

With reducing working hours and shift patterns becoming more common, there is a move from individual doctor patient care provision to team based care provision. Exchange of information between team members to allow safe and smooth continuity of care, is thus essential.

As a doctor you may handover patients to other doctors during normal working hours or when on call. You may also have to pass information to other healthcare staff such as anaesthetic recovery staff or nursing staff. Handovers may occur in community or hospital environments, in the Emergency Department, ward, post-surgery recovery room, or intensive care. Studies evaluating handover practises have shown deficiencies, often being non-structured and prone to errors [28–32].

Handover is not simply about passing a list of patients with their relevant clinical information and outstanding tasks. Efficient handover allows:

- Communication of concerns of the outgoing team.
- Communication of anticipated problems that the incoming team may face.
- Clear identification of those patients that are unwell and who need prompt attention.
- Information to allow prioritisation of tasks by the incoming team.

The exact handover process may vary according to the context in which you practise, or local system and organisation practicalities. Nevertheless, the following communication factors, based on guidance by the British and Australian Medical Associations, may improve your handover efficiency [27, 33]:

- Allow sufficient, uninterrupted time for handover. Avoid, short, rushed, verbal, corridor handovers.
- All stakeholders should be present, both with regards breadth of professionals' skills and seniority of such professionals.
- Include patients in hospital but also patients that have been referred and are still to be seen and assessed.
- Handover full details of patients, including location.
- Pass clinical information about patients in a structured way.
- Highlight your concerns.
- Highlight those tasks that need prompt attention.

A checklist system, written or electronic, which ensures confidentiality but also easy access to incoming and outgoing teams, may facilitate transfer of information in a structured manner. iSoBAR, a handover checklist, developed at the Royal Perth Hospital in Australia, and based on the SBAR tool, may facilitate handovers. It describes [34]:

i-dentify your self and patient
S-ituation
o-bservations
B-ackground
A-greed plan
R-ead back – to ensure proper receipt of information and strengthen
accountability.

Written Communication

> The ability to simplify means to eliminate the unnecessary so that the necessary may speak
>   Hans Hofmann [1]

Documentation of interactions with patients or other actions that involve patients' care, forms a substantial component of a doctor's work practise. Such documentation may involve making records of patients' assessments in the community, the Emergency Department, wards, or out-patient clinics. Documentation may involve making records of surgical procedures in theatres, making records of discussions with other colleagues, recording discussions with patients or relatives.

You may find yourself wondering why you spend lots and lots of time recording what has taken place, rather than actually doing things. But why is documentation so important?

- It allows you to look back to see how a patient's condition was at a particular time, and hence assess whether the condition has since changed.
- Continuity of care – allows another carer to pick up where you left things, when you are not present in person.
- Legal reasons – things may go wrong, patients may complain, you may need to refer back to see what actually took place. An action not documented may, in some legal systems, be considered as not to have taken place.
- Accurate documentation of delivered treatment may ensure proper remuneration of your institution. Remuneration may be based on procedures performed, diagnoses made, or patients' co-morbidities. This information must be recorded in order to be accounted for.
- The information you record may provide the tool of subsequent research or audits.

In documenting patients' assessments in medical charts there are certain principles to follow. Consider:

- Be thorough, yet succinct. Like in verbal presentations, highlight the important and relevant points, when documenting. It may be that you have to record initially a clinical assessment which is pages long. Do so, but also add a summary which can be referred to clearly and quickly.
- Have a systematic way to ensure that documentations are presented in a logical, easily followed manner. SBAR and SOAP, or your own modifications of these, could be used.
- Clearly sign and print your name at the end of any entries, so someone looking at the entry can identify who you are. A name stamp may help in a busy environment.
- If documenting on behalf of others, like a clinical review by a senior, make that clear.
- Date and time any entries, so it is clear as to when they happened.
- If hand written, use legible writing. What is the scope of writing if no-one can read it? If you can not read what you wrote, it is unlikely others will be able to do so.

Filling Forms

Whether written or electronic, forms are on the rise. No matter how daunting forms seem to be they are a way of communication, and should be treated like that. Forms may be used in requesting assessment by other teams, requesting physiotherapy or orthotics input, requesting tests or investigations. Consider forms not as another formidable task but as a way of standardising, and enhancing communication. Consider forms as a way of filling gaps of communication where those exist. Look at forms as the means of reminding you what information you need to provide. In completing forms several additional principles may apply:

- Check that the patient details are correct, and their contact details are up to date. What is their preferred contact means? Are they planning to be away?
- Give sufficient information and clearly state what you are asking for, yet be succinct so the message is not lost in reams of information.
- Have a structure in providing information. This may already be pre-set by the form's format, or you may have to determine what structure to adopt.
- Do not sign forms which are not completed, forms which do not have the patient's details on. What if the wrong name sticker is put on after you sign it? What if the wrong information is filled?
- Avoid leaving parts unfilled. If not relevant state that, rather than leaving it blank.
- Investigation request forms – state what investigation you are asking for, and the reason why you are asking this. Give sufficient clinical information to justify your request, but also to allow the receiver to appreciate what question you aim to answer. It maybe that in addition to all the rheumatology tests you are asking for there is another one that the lab can add, to further help you reach a diagnosis. The radiographer may be able to adjust the view of taking the requested radiograph, to help answer your specific question. It maybe that the radiologist can suggest that a computerised tomography (CT) scan is better than a magnetic resonance imaging (MRI) scan to look for fracture union. In addition to routine nerve tests the neurophysiologist may be able to add more complex EMG studies, to help diagnose the cause of newly onset neurological symptoms.

Discharge Summaries

A discharge summary may be considered as a statement created about a patient, upon discharge from a medical institution. Discharge summaries may be aimed at the doctor that will be looking after the patient in the community or in another institution, and aim to communicate the:

- Reasons for admission.
- Diagnosis or medical condition treated.

- Events that took place during the admission (treatment administered, tests performed, outcomes of investigations).
- Change in patient's condition.
- State of patient upon discharge.
- Post discharge plans or instructions for required actions (social input or house adjustments, physiotherapy, need for wound dressings, suture removals, mobilisation status, follow up appointments, referrals to other specialists, monitoring, further tests to be performed).
- Take away medications and the duration of prescription.

If looking after many patients in a ward or working in an environment with a high patient turnover (such as in day case surgical department), completing discharge summaries may provide a substantial workload. Nevertheless, discharge summaries must be given the time needed, as they form a vital piece of communication in ensuring continuity of care.

It is always a balance between giving sufficient information, but at the same time avoiding too much information, which may be time consuming, and fails to deliver a clear message. Put yourself in the receiver's shoes, and consider what information would you have liked to receive. Avoid abbreviations that are often used in a hospital environment but may be difficult to interpret by those practising in the community. A template, designed by your self or your institution, tailored to your specialty and the conditions you are dealing with, may improve efficiency whilst ensuring adequacy of transmitted information.

Referral Letters

Referral letters allow the transmission of information between healthcare professionals, and the request of input of one professional from another. The information you provide in a referral letter is vital in guiding the receiver as how to triage the patient, and prioritise with regards the timing of seeing a patient. The referral letter may be the only information available at the time of consultation, on which the assessor has to rely. Yet the quality of referral letters may not meet expected standards [35].

Referrals to other doctors or other health care professionals, may be in the form of structured forms, or self constructed letters. Whatever the format consider including:

- Patient's name and up to date contact details.
- Your details and address, date of letter.
- Whom you are addressing it to; a specific person, or a specific department? If referring a patient to a department rather than person the next available specialist could deal with it, which may influence waiting times.
- Reason for referral – to assess patient, give a further opinion, take over, discuss management options, treat, investigate.

- Urgency of request – routine, soon, urgent.
- Presenting complaint.
- Relevant previous medical history.
- Other important clinical history – allergies.
- Medications.
- Investigations and results.
- Up to date treatment for the condition and its response.
- Inform of any special circumstances, such as need for transport, need of interpreter.

If a test has been done that will aid in assessment, ensure that the full results will be available at the time of consultation. Your interpretation of results may not suffice. The specialist may need to look at the original scans or the spirometry results in person. This may save the patient back and forth appointments.

Clinic Consultation Letters

For patients seen in outpatients, clinic letters are often constructed as a response to the referrer, and aim to inform the referrer of the consultation events. In addition, they provide a record that you can refer to later on, if the patient were to come back. Whether hand written, typed, or in electronic form, consultation letters are vital communication and documentation tools.

As when writing referral letters, ensure that the details of the patient, originator and receiver, and the date of consultation are clearly stated. The letter format may vary according to your specialty, but an acceptable format is to give a short, easily read summary of the main message, at the top of the letter (Fig. 3.1). This may include the diagnosis or presenting symptoms, date at which diagnosis was made or date of onset of symptoms, and further plan (such as follow up arrangements, referral for investigations). You may then present the remaining letter, using the following sub-headings:

- Presenting complaint.
- Findings on clinical examination.
- Investigations and results.
- Impression/opinion regarding diagnosis.
- Plans for further treatment.
- Requests to referrer for further action.
- Outcome of consultation – discharged, follow up arrangements, referred to other specialty.
- Additional information to remind you or inform others copied in letter– such as patient needs to come back with translator present, patient listed for surgery and will need specialist equipment.

To: Dr………..

Patient's Name:………..
Date of birth:…………..

Diagnosis:…………………..
Date of onset of symptoms:…………..
Procedure:……………..
Plan:…………………

Many thanks for referring this patient,

who presents with a 4 month history of symptoms of
……………………………………………………………….

On examination clinical signs ………………….…………….
………………………………………………………………..

Investigations have shown
…………………………………………………………..

My working diagnosis is that of……………and my plan is
to……………………………………………………………..

I would be grateful if you could recheck the full blood
count…………………………………………………………….

Patient will be seen back in clinic in 4 weeks.

                                                                 Yours sincerely,

Fig. 3.1 Proposed out-patient clinic letter template

Maintain a structure to your letters, rather than going back and forth, mixing symptoms with signs and investigations.

You may find that in the end of consultation you need to inform not only the referrer, but also other professionals, with regards the consultation. Copy the letter to those too. If needed to ask another professional for input, based on that consultation, rather than writing a completely new letter from scratch, consider sending a shorter letter with your specific request, and attaching a copy of your main clinic letter to it.

Phoning

First learn the meaning of what you say, and then speak

Epictetus [1]

You may ring a colleague or other professional to ask for advice, receive or pass information, discuss a patient or a situation, request a patient's assessment, or ask for an investigation to be performed. Before you pick up the phone, spend some time planning the conversation ahead. Make sure you are in an environment where you can hear well and you are unlikely to be interrupted.

Before you lift up the phone consider:

- Why you are ringing.
- What specific answer or outcome you want to achieve.
- Do you have at hand all the details you may need? What might the other person ask, and do you have those answers?
- Have a system in presenting patients over the phone; SBAR and SOAP may once again help.
- Rehearse in your mind, or on paper, what you plan to say. Rehearse as how you will present the patient, or how you could describe a radiograph over the phone.

When you ring:

- Speak slowly and clearly.
- Ask other caller to speak slowly.
- Clearly state who you are.
- Check the caller's identity.
- Ask if they are able to speak.
- State clearly at the beginning the reason for ringing. Are you asking for advice, are you asking for a review of a patient, do you have a plan and you are simply informing your senior of your forthcoming actions, are you asking for an urgent test, are you asking for an action such as taking the patient to theatre for emergency surgery?
- Thank the caller at the end and make a record of the conversation in the notes.

Similar principles apply if you are responding to a phone call. Pay particular attention as to whether you are really sure who the caller is, to avoid breaching confidentiality. If unsure offer to ring the caller back.

Emailing

Words are only painted fire; a look is the fire itself

Mark Twain [1]

Emailing is part of modern life. No more need to wait for the postman, conversations in almost real time, live communications on the laptop, tablet, phone. Unlike verbal communication, emails provide time to digest the information you receive and consider your reply, yet give the option of a much faster response than traditional letters. Treat emails with the respect that any other form of written communication deserves. Use the same principles of communication as when meeting someone in person.

In emailing you may consider:

- As in verbal communication, be polite and respectful. Consider the person behind the email, rather than the email itself. Email rage has no place.
- Use them sparingly. Is it better to email someone or meet them in person? Is it better to just pick the phone?
- Emails are just another form of communication. Should you be putting in an email what you would not consider appropriate to say in person?
- Emails lack body language, facial expression, and tone of voice. Take this into account as to how you phrase things. What you may consider as a sharp response, may be perceived as uncaring by others.
- Who do you need to copy in emails? Is it necessary to copy all those people? What effect will this have on the response you are seeking from the email receiver? Are you copying someone to ask for action, to inform, or simply to create impressions and gather support? Should you be Bccing (blindly copying) if all should be open and transparent?
- If you want your email to be read only by its recipient, naming it "strictly confidential", or "just for you", may not suffice. Emails like letters may go astray. Is there information there that can not be shared? If you really would not like what you write to be seen by others, may be the safest option is not to write it at all.
- Reply promptly to your emails. Even if you can not give an immediate answer, acknowledge receipt as good manners. If someone spoke to you in the corridor, it is unlikely you would ignore them, why put off replying to that email?

Resendes et al. [36] evaluated the perceptions of surgical residents on received emails, at the McMaster University in Ontario, Canada. They assessed receivers with regards their preferred email formatting, their impression of the sender based on the email, and factors that influenced their response. Coloured backgrounds, difficult-to-read font, lack of a subject heading, opening salutations without using the recipient's name, or use of no salutation, were all negatively endorsed. Senders of negatively perceived e-mails were considered inefficient, unprofessional and irritating. Senders of positively perceived emails were more likely to be considered professional, pleasant, and kind. Participants were almost threefold more likely to respond immediately to emails they considered favourable, as compared to those they disliked.

Medical Reporting

Sick Leave/Fit Notes

Depending on where you practise, you may be asked to give a note to recommend whether a patient should refrain from work, or restrict their work activities, due to a particular medical condition. In completing such a note follow the law of the land, and your regulatory body advice, but you may consider the following:

- Inability to work may be because:
    - Certain activities would worsen an underlying medical condition (such as lifting heavy weights following an acute disc prolapse).
    - The symptoms of an underlying condition makes it difficult to carry certain tasks (back pain from disc prolapse makes it difficult to lift weights).
    - Inability to get to and from work (can not sit in bus too long or climb stairs due to back pain).
    - Returning to work may be unsafe (replacing tiles on a garage roof whilst getting intermittent episodes of sharp back pain).

State as to what the reasoning is for advising to avoid work. Consider:
- One may be able to work without being in perfect health. One may work without having to perform maximum duties.
- Check with patient as how much information they consent to providing with regards their condition. Ensure no breach of confidentiality.
- Describe the condition in plain language, avoiding technical terms.
- Be accurate as to dating; the date you are assessing the patient, versus the date you signed the sick note, versus the date from which patient may not have been able to work from (such as when patient stumbled and broke both ankles).
- Be specific in your instructions with regards complete absence from work, gradual return to work, ability to perform only certain activities.
- You may be able to advice about amending one's work duties, working hours, or workplace environment, to facilitate earlier return to work.
- If you are not familiar exactly with what the patient's job entails (as it is likely to be in many cases), state what activities, that could worsen the medical condition, should be avoided.

In writing a report to an employer with regards ability of an individual to work Cott and Goldeber [37] recommend answering five crucial questions, that will give clear guidance as to one's condition:

1. Is there a definitive diagnosis to explain complaints and symptoms?
2. Has optimal medical treatment been administered?
3. What irreducible limitations are imposed by the condition?
4. Are there any contraindications imposed by the condition? Distinguish between "hurt" and "harm", the latter being due to placing the individual at safety risk or exacerbating the condition.

5. Is the condition temporary or permanent? If temporary what is the time frame of recovery, and if permanent or progressive what is its likely route?

Statements, Medical Reports, Insurance Forms

You may be asked to provide a note informing a third party as to the medical condition of a patient, for insurance or other purposes. Consider the following;

- Obtain consent from patient as to what information you are allowed to share.
- Check with patient if they want to see a copy of you report, prior to sending it through.
- State your relation and details of contact with patient.
- State the facts you know or you directly witnessed.
- If you are simply reporting facts stated by others (such as information provided by patient collected through another doctors clerking), say so.
- Be accurate with dates.
- Avoid personal interpretations of events or assumptions.
- Use simple terms, easy for a lay person to understand.

Consenting

Informed consent is the process of obtaining permission for conducting an intervention on an individual. This may be an invasive or non-invasive procedure, other treatment, or participation in a research trial. Consent should be given voluntarily by an adequately informed individual, who is able to do so. Consent may be written or verbal. If obtaining consent follow the laws of the land and rules of your regulatory body. In England there is no statute setting out the principles of consent. However, it has been established, through case law, that touching a patient without valid consent may constitute a civil or criminal offence or even battery [38].

Documentation of the consent process records the explanation of the proposed procedure to a patient and the patient's agreement. It includes:

- A description of the proposed intervention.
- Intended benefits of the intervention.
- Risks the procedure may entail.
- Additional interventions that may become necessary.
- Specifies the identity, professional title, or seniority of the healthcare professional carrying out the intervention.

In consenting it is necessary to recognise what constitutes competency for consenting, who can seek consent, and what risks must be explained. Such factors may vary from country to country. In the United Kingdom (UK) guidelines by the Department of Health [29] state that:

1. As per the Mental capacity Act [39] "a person lacks capacity if: they have an impairment of disturbance (for example a disability, condition or trauma or the effect of drugs or alcohol) that affects the way their mind or brain works, and that impairment or disturbance means that they are unable to make a specific decision at the time it needs to be made".
2. General Medical Council guidance [40] states that the person obtaining consent should be appropriately trained and qualified. The person obtaining consent should have adequate knowledge of the proposed procedure and should understand the procedure risks, to provide any necessary explanation.
3. It is recommended that any significant risks should be explained to the patient, even if these are rare. This follows a case law judgement (Chester v Afshar) [41]. In that case the patient was not informed with regards the risk of cauda equina in spinal surgery, and was left partially paralysed following the procedure. Hence, it was held that failure to warn a patient of a risk related to surgery, no matter how rare that may be, could deny a patient the ability to make a fully informed decision.

Documentation of the consent process may be achieved through pre-designed structured consent forms. Documentation provides a record of the consent process, but also helps communicating the consent process to others involved in a patient's care. In completing a consent form, several principles may apply:

- Follow the rules of your institution or medical authority with regards using provided pre-designed forms.
- If there are no pre-designed forms, or those provided do not allow for the essential information to be recorded, make a note in the patient's records, documenting the consent process.
- Eligibility in completing consent forms is vital, as these will be checked by various staff (such as at various stages on the way to the operating room).
- Avoid abbreviations that may confuse the reader. Use capital letters where necessary to make reading easier.
- Be clear as to who can sign a consent form, as per patient's age, or next of kin. If uncertain, check with your seniors, or the legal department of your institution.
- Complete such forms well in advance of the intervention, thus giving adequate time to the patient to consider facts and change mind is necessary.
- Give a copy of the signed consent form to the patient.

Writing a Business Case

The person who says it cannot be done should not interrupt the person who is doing it
Chinese proverb [1]

"Dragon's Den" is a popular television series screened by the British Broadcasting Corporation (BBC). In this, entrepreneurs present a new product or invention to a group of successful millionaires, asking them for money and networking to help build their business [42]. Successful investment bids rely on having a novel, likely desirable product, but also upon an outstanding, well thought presentation, that takes into account what the new product is, why it is needed, the cost implications, and the risks of the business proposal.

As doctors we often want to introduce a new service or improve an existing one, to advance care quality. Such changes may have substantial financial and resource implications. Hence, thorough justification for such changes is warranted.

A business plan can allow you to put such a case forwards to the relevant authorities of your institution or external bodies, asking for their support. Even if you are self employed, and the final decision relies upon yourself, a business plan may help put structure to your thoughts, to fully evaluate your ideas before you proceed.

Writing a business case is an attempt to put in a clear, simplified way, a proposal with its potential benefits, associated implications and risks. The following is a suggested format for writing a business plan:

1. Summary of the proposal.
2. Background – what the clinical problem is, what the current status is, why there is a need for change.
3. Describe the proposed implementation.
4. Potential benefits of new implementation.
5. Risks of implementation.
6. Alternatives – doing nothing, other options, what their benefits and risks are, how they compare with your preferred proposal.
7. Resource and costs implications of proposal.
8. Timescales of introduction, achieving improvement.
9. Means of assessing outcomes of new proposal.
10. Alternative plans in place.
11. Conclusions.
12. Supporting references from published literature.
13. Additional information (details of a new technology, learning lessons from other institution implementing proposal).

Breaking Bad News

As a doctor you may find your self in a position of having to communicate bad news to a patient, or patient's relatives. In a managerial position you may have to communicate bad news to colleagues, peers, juniors, or other staff. You may be assessed in communicating bad news as part of a postgraduate examination, or in attending an interview for a new post.

Breaking bad news is a difficult, challenging, uncomfortable task, often associated with high emotions. The skill of communicating bad news is hence one to be developed and mastered. In doing so consider the following:

- Plan what you will say and how you will say it. Rehearse if necessary.
- Ensure the receiver will have someone to provide emotional support; a relative, friend, other staff member.
- Have a clear plan, to communicate what arrangements have been made for the future. Have a specific time plan. This plan may be for further investigations, specific treatment, specific referral to another specialist with time and date confirmed. Communicate this once you break the bad news. If necessary delay breaking the bad news until such a plan is in place.
- Use a venue where you can speak and be heard clearly, with no interruptions.
- Allocate sufficient time. Do not look or sound rushed.
- Break the news gently. Give cues as to what is coming, but avoid missing the message for the sake of breaking the news gradually.
- The message must be clear and definite, with no uncertainties as to what has been said. If needed, try and repeat the message in different verbal forms.
- Use plain language, avoid medical or managerial jargons.
- Enquire about the receiver's understanding of your message.
- Give time for the news to sink in, and give the opportunity to be asked questions.
- Offer to come back and discuss matters further.

References

1. Famous Quotes at BrainyQuote. www.brainyquote.com. Accessed on 23 Sept 14.
2. Kahn MW. Etiquette-based medicine. N Engl J Med. 2008;358:1988–9.
3. Mehrabian A, Ferris SR. Inference of attitudes from nonverbal communication in two channels. J Consult Psychol. 1967;31(3):48–258.
4. Mehrabian A, Wiener M. Decoding of inconsistent communications. J Pers Soc Psychol. 1967;6:109–14.
5. Mehrabian A. Silent messages. Belmont: Wadsworth; 1971.
6. Guerrero LK, Andersen PA, Afifi WA. Close encounters: communication in relationships. 3rd ed. California, USA: SAGE Publications, Inc.; 2010.
7. Burgoon JK, Hale JL. The fundamental topic of relational communication. Commun Monogr. 1984;51:193–214.
8. Step MM, Rose JH, Albert JM, Cheruvu VK, Siminoff LA. Modelling patient-centered communication: oncologist relational communication and patient communication involvement in breast cancer adjuvant therapy decision-making. Patient Educ Couns. 2009;77(3):369–781.
9. Shay LA, Dumenci L, Siminoff LA, Flocke SA, Lafata JE. Factors associated with patient reports of positive physician relational communication. Patient Educ Couns. 2012;89(1):96–101.
10. Orioles A, Miller VA, Kersun LS, Ingram M, Morrison WE. "To be a phenomenal doctor you have to be the whole package": physicians' interpersonal behaviors during difficult conversations in pediatrics. J Palliat Med. 2013;16(8):929–33.
11. Profiles in improvement. Doug Bonacum of Kaiser Permanente. Institute for Healthcare Improvement; 2008. http://www.ihi.org/knowledge/Pages/AudioandVideo/ProfilesinImprovementDougBonacumofKaiserPermanente.aspx. Accessed 25 Sept 14.
12. Weed LL. Medical records, medical education, and patient care: the problem-oriented medical record as a basic tool. Cleveland: Case Western Reserve University; 1970.
13. Joint Commission on Accreditation of Healthcare Organizations. Sentinel event statistics data – root causes by event type (2004–2013). http://www.jointcommission.org. Accessed 18 Aug 14.
14. Advanced life support. Resuscitation Council (UK), London, UK. 6th ed. 2011.
15. ATLS: Advanced Trauma Life Support for Doctors (Student course manual). American College of Surgeons. 8th ed. Chicago, USA: American College of Surgeons; 2008. ISBN-10: 1880696312.
16. WHO surgical safety checklist and implementation manual. http://www.who.int/patientsafety/safesurgery/ss_checklist/en/. Accessed on 20 Sept 14.
17. Makary MA, Holzmueller CG, Thompson D, Rowen L, Heitmiller ES, Maley WR, Black JH, Stegner K, Freischlag JA, Ulatowski JA, Pronovost PJ. Operating room briefings: working on the same page. Jt Comm J Qual Patient Saf. 2006;32(6):351–5.
18. AirDisaster. Com: Investigation: United Airlines Flight 173. www.airdisaster.com. Accessed on 1 Sept 14.
19. Helmreich RL, Merritt AC, Wilhelm JA. The evolution of crew resource management training in commercial aviation. Int J Aviat Psychol. 1999;9:19–32.
20. Cooper GE, White MD, Lauber JK, editors. Resource management on the flight deck: Proceedings of a NASA/Industry workshop held at San Francisco, California, June 26–28, 1979. NASA Conference Publication 2120, Mar 1980.
21. Oriol MD. Crew resource management: applications in healthcare organizations. J Nurs Adm. 2006;36:402–6.
22. Bhangu A, Bhangu S, Stevenson J, Bowley DM. Lessons for surgeons in the final moments of Air France Flight 447. World J Surg. 2013;37(6):1185–92.
23. Agency for Healthcare Research and Quality. http://teamstepps.ahrq.gov/. Accessed on 25 Sept 14.
24. Hopkins J. The human factor: the two challenge rule. 2013. http://www.flyingmag.com. Accessed on 25 Sept 14.

25. Hopkins J. President of the Error Prevention Institute, Inc. Personal communication. Personal communication via email, 14 Aug 14.
26. Committee on Quality of Health Care in America, Institute of Medicine, et al. To err is human. In: Kohn LT, Corrigan JM, Donaldson MS, editors. Building a safer health system. Washington, DC: National Academy Press; 2000. ISBN 10: 0309261740.
27. BMA, Junior Doctors Committee, National Patient Safety Agency, NHS Modernisation Agency. Safe handover: safe patients. Guidance on clinical handover for clinicians and managers. London: BMA; 2005.
28. Ferran NA, Metcalfe AJ, O'Doherty D. Standardised proformas improve patient handover: audit of trauma handover practice. Patient Saf Surg. 2008;2:24.
29. Ilan R, LeBaron CD, Christianson MK, Heyland DK, Day A, Cohen MD. Handover patterns: an observational study of critical care physicians. BMC Health Serv Res. 2012;12:11. doi:10.1186/1472-6963-12-11.
30. Shafiq-ur-Rehman, Mehmood S, Ahmed J, Razzaq MH, Khan S, Perry EP. Surgical handover in an era of reduced working hours: an audit of current practice. J Coll Physicians Surg Pak. 2012;22(6):385–8.
31. Siddiqui N, Arzola C, Iqbal M, Sritharan K, Guerina L, Chung F, Friedman Z. Deficits in information transfer between anaesthesiologist and postanaesthesia care unit staff: an analysis of patient handover. Eur J Anaesthesiol. 2012;29(9):438–45.
32. Kalkman CJ. Handover in the perioperative care process. Curr Opin Anaesthesiol. 2010;23(6):749–53.
33. Australian Medical Association. Safe handover: safe patients. Guidance on clinical handover for clinicians and managers. Canberra: AMA; 2006. http://www.ama.com.au. Accessed 23/9/14.
34. Porteous JM, Stewart-Wynne EG, Connolly M, Crommelin PF. iSoBAR–a concept and handover checklist: the national clinical handover initiative. Med J Aust. 2009;190(11):S152–6.
35. Jiwa M, Coleman M, McKinley R. Measuring the quality of referral letters about patients with upper gastrointestinal symptoms. Postgrad Med J. 2005;81(957):467–9.
36. Resendes S, Ramanan T, Park A, Petrisor B, Bhandari M. Send it: study of e-mail etiquette and notions from doctors in training. J Surg Educ. 2012;69(3):393–403.
37. Cott A, Goldberg WM. Doctors' notes to employers and insurers. Can Fam Physician. 1985;31:1919–25.
38. Department of Health. Reference guide to consent for examination or treatment. 2nd ed. 2009. www.dh.gov.uk/consent. Accessed on 23 Sept 14.
39. Mental Capacity Act 2005 – Legislation.gov.uk www.legislation.gov.uk.
40. Consent: patients and doctors making decisions together. London: GMC; 2008. www.gmc-uk.org/guidance.
41. Judgments – Chester (Respondent) v. Afshar (Appellant). [2004] UKHL 41 http://www.publications.parliament.uk/pa/ld200304/ldjudgmt/jd041014/cheste-1.htm. Accessed 25 Sept 14.
42. BBC Two –Dragons' Den. www.bbc.co.uk/programmes. Accessed 23 Sept 14.

Chapter 4
Professionalism

Professionalism refers to the ability to work and behave in a manner that upholds the standards required and set by one's profession.

Several definitions of medical professionalism have been put forwards. The Royal College of Physicians of London defined professionalism as a set of values, behaviours and relationships that forms the basis of the trust that the public has in doctors [1]. David Stern, Professor of Medicine of the University of Michigan, United States of America (USA), and editor of the book "Measuring Medical Professionalism", describes excellence, accountability, altruism and humanism as the four central principles of medical professionalism [2]. Professor Tim Wilkinson, director of the Faculty of Medicine at the University of Otago, New Zealand, and his colleagues, defined professionalism as consisting of adherence to ethical practise (honesty, integrity), effective interactions with patients (empathy, respect), effective interaction with other healthcare workers (team work), reliability (accountability), and commitment to continuous self improvement (constant learning) [3].

Professionalism may be taught, but may also be acquired through observation of behaviours of those around us, including juniors, peers, seniors, and role models. Professionalism may also be developed through the ongoing reflection of our interactions with other healthcare workers, patients and relatives.

Certain professional conducts may be unique to Medicine, but others may be applied to a wide range of professions. This chapter addresses several behaviours which may affect your professional image. It is not meant to be an exhaustive list but a presentation of commonly encountered actions, which may shape one's professional standing.

© Springer International Publishing Switzerland 2015
C. Panayiotou Charalambous, *Career Skills for Doctors*,
DOI 10.1007/978-3-319-13479-6_4

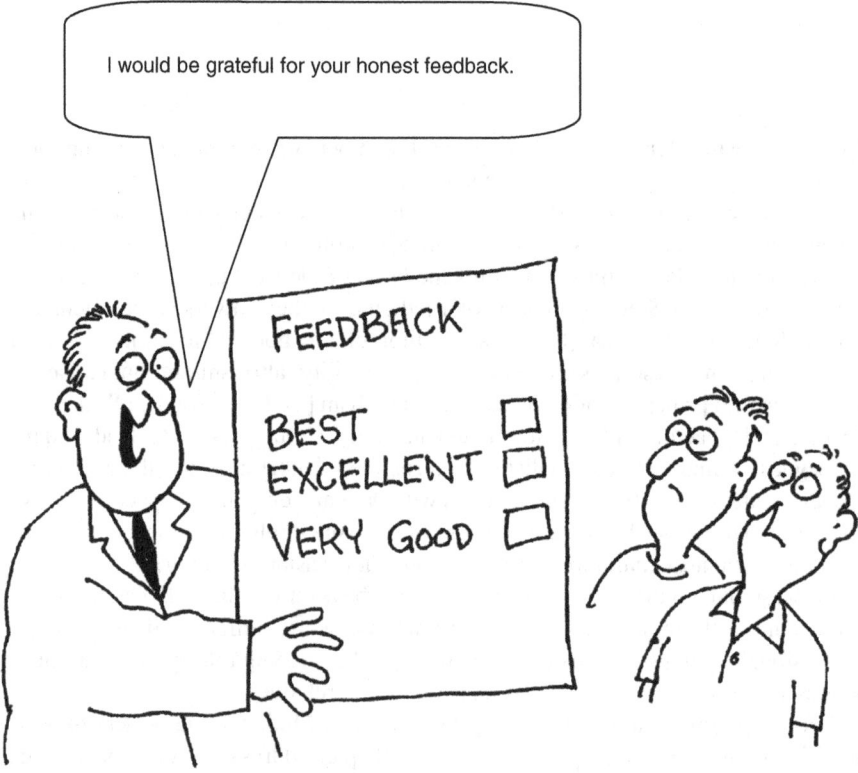

Respect All Staff, Medical and Non-medical Alike

Respect a man, and he will do all the more

John Wooden [4]

There is little scope in being respectful, friendly, and obedient, to your immediate seniors and other medical staff, yet being abrupt and dismissive of the ward clerk, the receptionist, the porter, the nurse. Hospitals, like any other organisation, rely not only on those at the top, but also on those lower down, the many unsung heroes.

How fast your operating theatre list runs, may depend on how quickly the porter brings the next patient from ward. How smoothly your clinic runs, may depend on how quickly the receptionist checks in patients. Your assessment of a new ward patient may rely on the ward clerk promptly locating and bringing you the patient's previous records.

If you are not respectful to other staff, if you are rude or harsh, the word goes round and your seniors may soon find out. Those you are rude to may complain and then there may be trouble.

A well known surgeon, Lord Ara Darzi, Professor of Surgery at St Mary's hospital in London, UK, recalls going undercover, as a hospital porter doing a night shift [5]:

> ...the third year medical student looked right through me as he commanded, "You grab the feet and pull . .. then go up to the ward and bring down the next patient, and hurry. . . it's because of you this list is running behind." He certainly put me in my place...The moment I put on the uniform and walked into theatres to transfer my first patient of the shift I effectively disappeared from the view of my medical colleagues and now irreverent students.... my peers and students would no longer look me in the eyes, and I at once felt dismembered from the close knit clinical team,

whilst the next morning, when back as a surgeon:

> On arrival at theatre, now dressed in scrubs and clearly identifiable as a surgeon ready to operate, I received quite a different welcome from that I had only hours before.

Being respectful to others and recognising their contribution, is not only the noble thing to do. It helps get the most out of all, encourages them to give their best self. By bringing all staff together, your patients will get the best deal.

Respect Colleagues, Juniors and Seniors Alike

This is the first test of a gentleman: his respect for those who can be of no possible value
to him

William Lyon Phelps [4]

Respect your colleagues whether of the same level, junior or senior, whether or not you are directly answerable or accountable to them. Mutual respect forms the basis of team work and professional cooperation.

Your newly started juniors may not be very sleek at cannulation, not very quick at taking medical histories, may need assistance for urinary catheterisation, may have never plastered an ankle before, or may have just asked a question they ought to already know the answer to. Show patience, understanding, offer guidance and support. Wisdom, knowledge and slickness come with experience, with years of training and learning. After all, it may not be long since you were junior. Treat others as you would have liked to be treated at that level. You might have been much brighter, flying high when at their stage, but still provide all necessary help.

Respect not only your immediate seniors and colleagues but also those you do not usually work with, or are not directly answerable to. A senior from a different specialty may visit your ward to see an outlier. Even though that senior is not involved in your training, not someone to get a future reference from, offer assistance if you can. In a busy environment, such gesture may reflect well on yourself, your ward, your team, your specialty. And who knows, it may be that senior and your boss are having lunch later on. A senior from a different specialty may try to refer you a patient for assessment and admission. You may disagree with the need for the referral. Rather than bluntly refusing and rudely arguing, make alternative suggestions in a polite, diplomatic way. If there is still disparity of views, offer to discuss this with your own senior to get back with an answer. You can thus stand your ground, whilst offering a solution, and diffusing rather than escalating a tense situation. Picking fights with those at a higher level is not necessarily a sign of strength, a sign that you can punch above your weight. Being respectful in difficult times is more of a sign of strength.

Be Assertive

There is nothing intelligent about not standing up for yourself. You may not win every battle. However, everyone will at least know what you stood for—YOU

Shannon Alder [4]

In a healthy workplace mutual respect is essential. You are expected to respect others yet expect the same respect back. An environment whereby some workers are passive and simply follow the demands of others is not healthy. Neither is an environment whereby some workers get their way through aggressiveness and constant confrontation. You are not at work to simply please everyone else or for everyone else simply to please you. Assertion is described by Ken and Kate Back in their book "Assertiveness at Work" as "Standing up for your own rights in such a way that you do not violate another person's rights" and "Expressing your needs, wants, opinions, feelings, and beliefs in direct, honest and appropriate ways" [6].

Assertion refers to resisting being taken advantage of, yet not being pushy to others. It refers to saying "no" and refusing tasks you are not meant to do. The ten rules of assertion described by Chris Williams [7], Senior lecturer at the Department of Psychological Medicine of the University of Glasgow, UK, are:

1. Respect thyself.
2. Recognise your individual needs.
3. Use clear "I" statements to describe your feelings and thoughts.
4. Recognise you are allowed to make mistakes.
5. Recognise you can change your mind if you wish.
6. Ask to think over a request, rather than giving an immediate answer.
7. Enjoy your successes and wins.
8. Ask for what you want, rather than hoping others will notice what you are after.
9. Appreciate you are not responsible for how other individuals behave.
10. Support the right of being assertive.

As in other environments, assertion is often needed in the healthcare workplace:

- It maybe that a peer trainee keeps joining your operating list, hampering your training opportunities.
- It maybe colleagues keep passing all their work to you, rather than finishing it themselves.
- It maybe your senior demands you help them in their private practise, on your day off.
- It maybe your junior keeps coming late, for the morning ward rounds.
- It maybe that you are repeatedly called to the ward for non-urgent tasks, and no justifiable reason.
- It maybe your weekly rota keeps changing at short notice, making it impossible to plan your social life.

Whatever your seniority or level of training, stand up for yourself, for your beliefs and profession.

Avoid Public Arguments

Arguments are to be avoided, they are always vulgar and often convincing

Oscar Wilde [4]

Avoid arguments in front of other staff, your juniors, your colleagues, your patients.

What would you think if on a social night out a couple start arguing in front of you? Would you try to work out who is right and who is wrong, or would you think they are both unwise, for not sorting their troubles at home?

What would the medical students or nurses think, if they see their ward doctors having a go at each other, in front of them? What would a patient or patient's relatives think, if they were observers of such argument? What would the juniors, nurses, managers, or other professionals think if they are copied in heated, impressively constructed, point scoring, email exchanges between peers or colleagues? Would one of the doctors score brownie points, or would they both look foolish? Would they look respectful, worthy of their title, position and profession, or would they simply give a bad impression? Would they stamp their authority, or look unable to control their behaviour and emotions?

Arguments do happen, and on occasions you may have a frank talk, a heated discussion, with a colleague or other staff. It may be better to try and have such discussions in private, behind closed doors, away from the pressure of the eyes and ears of all those around you. Sometimes, it is not what we say, but also in front of whom we say it, that matters. Discuss to resolve, to find a middle ground, and move on.

Do Not Make It Personal

Fights begin and end with handshakes

Cameron Conaway [4]

You may have frank discussions, heated exchanges, or even arguments with medical colleagues, or other staff. You may want to look forwards others keep looking in the past. You may disagree to how things should be done, have strong differences in opinion. You may be in the right, the others may be in the wrong, they may not want to reason, you may not be able to compromise.

You may prefer being ward based, others being attached to a single team. You may want to swap teams half way through the attachment, others may want to stay afoot. You may view a ward closure as loss of services, others as a cost efficiency move. You may see moving to 7 day working as a revolutionary step for care provision, others as an antisocial move. You may feel a foot abscess warrants vascular admission, others may consider it an orthopaedic condition. You may want more time to assess a patient prior to admission, others may be pressing you for an immediate decision. You may feel a CT scan is needed to help you reach a diagnosis, but the radiologist may feel it is not justifiable. You may feel that a specialist cardiology input is necessary, but your request is dismissed as non essential. You may feel that the appendicitis case should go first to theatre, but the orthopaedic surgeons may feel that the child with the nasty fracture should jump the queue.

Argue and fight your case, argue against what you disagree with. However, try to treat such arguments as a matter of different opinions rather than a matter of personalities. You are not arguing against the bearers of opposite views but against the views themselves. Heated discussions should not affect your relations with the other side, together you may work on.

Expect the Courtesy You Give

Remember, no one can make you feel inferior without your consent

Eleanor Roosevelt [4]

Be polite, courteous, respectful, and expect the same from others. If someone's tone of voice is intimidating, makes you feel uncomfortable, or they are rude, tell them that you can not accept such behaviour, and ask them to stop. They may be tired, overworked, overstressed. You may be junior, you may have just started your new post, you may be finding your feet, you may have overlooked a task, or you may have made an error. None of these can justify being shouted at, being talked down, being pushed around.

You are a doctor, you are a professional, and you are there to do your job at the best of your abilities. You are there to develop your skills, to learn and progress. You recognise and accept any mistakes or deficiencies, and you are prepared to learn from them. It is only right to demand the same courtesy and respect that you give others.

If the other person is not prepared to treat you as you treat them, escalate this to the appropriate authorities – your seniors, your clinical and educational supervisors, the personnel department. Aim to stop it early before it gets out of control, before it gets you down.

Aim for Functional Relationships

You have to get along with people, but you also have to recognize that the strength of a team is different people with different perspectives and different personalities

Steve Case [4]

Differences of opinions with other staff, may not be short lived, but may be part of long term problematic relationships. Difficult relationships may arise for various reasons, including conflicting personalities, conflicting priorities, competition for resources, and competition for personal gain or progress. Being able to deal effectively with such difficult relationships is a sign of professionalism, and an important skill to develop. If not dealt with successfully, difficult relationships may prove disruptive to the workplace, and may lead to overwhelming anxiety and distress to those involved.

Psychiatrists Anthony Garelick and Leonard Fagin, in their article "Doctor to doctor: getting on with colleagues", describe their golden rules in dealing with difficult relationships [8]:

- Empathise with the other party. Try to see their point of view.
- Consider a quiet chat, or informal discussion, to explore and resolve differences.
- Seek advice from a trustworthy, impartial colleague.
- Be prepared to use formal structures and processes if differences become disruptive and if informal discussions prove fruitless. Such processes may be internal or external to your organisation. Know what supporting services are available.
- Face the problem rather than avoiding it. Deal with it early, before it gets out of control.
- Learn from any mistakes you made. Reflect on your behaviours and approach.

It is important to recognise that difficulties in getting on with colleagues and other staff, can exist as part of working life and that Medicine is not immune from these. It is also essential to recognise that not all relationships have to be perfect to be functional. We do not have to be best friends, or friends, at all, with other staff, for a working relationship to exist. Aim for a middle ground which can allow you to get on enough with others, to support a constructive relationship.

A unique situation of difficult relationships is that between a trainee and a trainer, where the differences in seniority and dependence of trainee on trainer for learning, development and career progression may complicate matters. When it comes to a trainer facing a difficult trainee, one may distinguish between behaviours which affect performance, and those that do not. The "managing under-performance" section of the management skills chapter, gives guidance on how to deal with under-performance. If behaviours are not affecting performance, the rules of working relationships may be employed.

Similarly, in dealing with a difficult trainer [9], one may apply the rules of working relationships:

- Is the trainer right? Is the behaviour of the trainer justified? Could you be in the wrong? Do you need help or support?
- Discuss with trainer in a polite and courteous matter. The trainer may not realise that their behaviour is offending.
- Seek advice from colleagues, other seniors, professional support bodies.
- Escalate, if discussion with trainer is not successful, or if it feels impossible for such discussion to take place. Escalate both with regards the workplace management ladder but also the training system ladder (local training tutor, head of specialty training, head of overall postgraduate training).
- Act early.

Get Involved in Good Politics

One of the penalties for refusing to participate in politics is that you end up being governed by your inferior

Plato [4]

Politics is defined as "the activities associated with the governance of a country or area, especially the debate between parties having power" [10].

You may feel like "I went into Medicine not politics, better leave politics to the politicians". Medicine is not only about looking after patients at the bedside, in the clinic or the operating room. It is also about the bigger picture, the system and structure in which healthcare is delivered, the availability, and allocation of resources. Some policies or decisions may initially look remote and not relevant to us, but may eventually filter down and have a direct effect on our day to day clinical practise.

Decisions may have to be made about the allocation of funding, staffing, and other resources in your hospital, city, region or country. Wards or hospitals may have to be shut, services slimmed down, sites merged. Your working terms and conditions may be under review, moving to shift work or 7 day working. Allocation of funding for research in your subspecialty may be under threat. Changes may be looming, with regards the length, structure, or aims of postgraduate training.

Keep an open ear, be aware of the current issues. Attend events and meetings to express your views, vote for representatives who stand up for your case and will fight for your beliefs, get involved in committees, try and influence the future from inside. Have an opinion and express it when asked or needed. Try to be a participant rather than a mere observer, bring ideas and make suggestions.

If you do not get involved in politics then politics will not involve you. Do you want to have a say or let others decide for you?

Avoid Bad Politics

Politics is the art of looking for trouble, finding it everywhere, diagnosing it incorrectly and applying the wrong remedies

Groucho Marx [4]

Politics may also be defined as "activities aimed at improving someone's status or increasing power within an organisation" [10].

Avoid pitiful politics. Avoid plots and intrigues, manipulative behaviours, fights for power and control, or hidden agendas, which may occur at workplaces. Avoid making your actions or beliefs the tool of getting at others. Be honest and straight in your beliefs, be clear about situations you do not like, but do not let these cloud your mind.

Who will gain the trust of others? The plotter who says one thing but has something else in mind, who tries to turn others against each other? Or the one who what you see is what you get, what you hear is what is meant, someone of high discretion and integrity? Avoid gossiping or speaking badly of others, your juniors, peers, or seniors. It does not reflect well on you. What you say may reach their ears; there may be lots of "well wishers" aiming to spread the word.

During your career progression or training, you may move from hospital to hospital, from department to department, spending only a short time in each of these. In medical organisations, like any workplace, staff may have arguments, feuds, big egos which may not compromise. If these do not directly affect you, avoid making them your business. You will not score many brownie points by taking sites. Many of those you see, or think are, arguing will be colleagues for many years, will have their ups and downs. You are there to be trained, look after patients, and develop your career.

Would you like to be remembered as someone who gave the best to their job, or as someone who was taking sides, speaking badly of people behind their backs, throwing oil in the fire? Even if you are driven into such situations, try to stay well out.

Agree in Advance

Good accounts make good friends

French proverb [11]

Agree in advance as to what the rules of engagement are so these are not questioned later. Avoid misunderstandings, avoid leaving issues un-clarified, and hoping for the best. Your perception of an arrangement may be different from that of other parties.

- You may be setting up a research project. Who will be doing what? Who will lead, who will follow? Who will be the first author, who will be last? What if someone does not complete the assigned task?
- You may have agreed to doing additional work or overtime. What will your exact duties be? What is the remuneration? Will you be paid by the hour or session? What if the session is cancelled, what if you finish early or overrun? Who will confirm how much time you worked? When will you be paid?
- You may swap your on call. When will it be paid back? What if your colleague changes post?
- You may be entitled 3 weeks of annual leave whilst rotating over three attachments. Can it all be taken in one post or does it have to be split?
- You may be asked to collect data for a departmental audit. Who is leading the audit? Will your work be acknowledged? Will you be one of the authors on any presentations or articles that arise?
- You may be given a post for a year to be reviewed at 6 months. What does this mean? Another interview? An informal chat? A formal assessment? Does it depend on day to day performance or do you have to pass an exam? By when will you know if you can stay on?
- You may get funding from industry, for a research project. Who will own the results? Will you be able to publish your outcomes no matter what the results are?

Make clear transparent agreements, rather than trying to sort matters out at a later stage. Know where you stand, before it is too late.

Speak Out

If you don't stand for something, you will fall for anything

Alexander Hamilton [12]

Speak out when things are not right. You are in a position of high responsibility, you are answerable, above all, to your patients. If things are not right, and patients are not getting a good deal, then say so.

It maybe patients in surgical wards can not receive prompt cardiology input. It maybe out of hours there is not sufficient senior support. It maybe patients are waiting too long for clinic appointments or surgery. It maybe patients can not be discharged for lack of social services. It maybe nursing care is not up to scratch. It maybe a colleague is under-performing.

Follow the formal procedures of your organisation or the procedures of the medical system you are practising in, to voice your concerns. This may involve communicating your concerns to your managers, your supervisors, your trainers, the overseeing medical body, the health care regulators. Explain the situation, the problems encountered, the difficulties faced. If not heard by those you initially approach, be prepared to take it further and speak out.

You may be worried about your job, the potential financial loss, the loss of colleagues' loyalty, the loss of your employer's support. But your main loyalty is towards your patients, your main duty of care is towards them. Sometimes we have to risk a lot, for what matters the most.

Complain Aiming for Change

I like to complain and do nothing to make things better

Kurt Cobain [4]

You may be unhappy about how the department is run, about your heavy workload, about the quality of projects you are asked to take, about the lack of support. In complaining consider the following:

- Be specific – for a problem to be identified, investigated, and resolved, the specifics of the issue must be clear. Be specific as to what you are complaining about, rather than generalise and group everyone the same. Is it fair to say that you do not have any senior support when on call, when actually you are having difficulty with only one senior to come and assess patients when needed? Is it right to complain that all juniors are work shy, when you only have in mind someone specific who spends most time in the coffee room? Is it fair to complain that the teaching program is substandard, when you actually could not follow only one specific lecture?
- Complain in a timely fashion – complain when problems arise. If you leave all to pile up, and simply give feedback at the end when you are ready to move on, how will things be improved? Will the person you are complaining about, recall those events to give a fair answer? Even though it may help future doctors, that may find themselves in that position, will it help you? Would it be right to complain at the end of your attachment that you did not manage to join the cardiology clinic, when you never raised it with your trainers prior to that? It may help others in the future, but your training opportunities may have already been lost.
- Complain to those who can achieve change – should you be complaining to the head of the training, if you have not raised those issues firstly with your trainer? Should you be complaining to the hospital chief, if you have not raised those problems within your department? Would it be right to report a trainee to their head of training for under-performance without firstly discussing the issues with the trainee? Raise your complains initially with the authorities which are at the frontline of addressing your worries. Give them an opportunity to respond, and if their actions do not suffice then take it further.
- If complaining about other staff, complain to their line manager. Inform your senior of the complaint, but note that your senior may not be able to directly influence the person you are complaining about.

Someone in high authority may know you, may be willing to support you, stand by you in times of need. However, how would it look if at the first sign of trouble, you turn to a higher authority for support?

Do Not Jump to Conclusions Easily

People who jump to conclusions rarely alight on them

Philip Guedalla [4]

Give an opinion taking into accounts all facts. A colleague may have made the wrong diagnosis, surgery performed by others may have led to complications, treatment may have been delayed. The patient, your juniors or colleagues, may seek your opinion as to whether things could have been done better. Could an alternative diagnosis have been reached, given the information available at the time? If the hip fracture were more rigidly fixed would it still have fallen apart? Were all those tests really essential or could treatment have been commenced earlier? Was the decision to proceed with cardiac surgery rather than stenting the correct one? Should the fracture have been fixed or should have it been left alone?

Give a truthful opinion after taking into account all available and necessary facts. Seek information and examine it carefully. If that means that you can not give an opinion because you do not know all the details of what took place, then say so. If it is hindsight that makes you wise, say so. If things could have been done better, if an obvious mistake took place, again say so. You might have done things differently, because your way of doing things is different. Nevertheless, if what was done, by someone else, was also an appropriate way of acting, then again say so, and make it clear.

Do not rush into condemning others, because you do not get on with them, or because doing so makes you look wiser and better. Similarly, do not rush to defend others, simply because they are close to you. Give an honest, fact based opinion. Give a view that you would be prepared to stand up for, and defend if the need arose. What you say is likely to be held tight, by those seeking your opinion.

Team Member

Individual commitment to a group effort – that is what makes a team work, a company work, a society work, a civilization work
                                                                        Vincent Lombard [13]

Being a member of a team, is a term you will hear about lots. It does not mean sacrifice self for team, put others above thy self. Instead, team working is about meeting your obligations and duties, sharing a common goal, and cooperating with others to achieve that goal. Restricted working hours, shift work, and fixed training commitments, may threaten the coherence and continuity of team work. However, certain behaviours may help you improve your team working performance:

- If you are going on annual leave or if away on teaching, have you made sufficient and robust arrangements to cover your duties? Will the colleague who agreed to cover your duties be truly around, or will they be on nights, or on call covering other wards? Have you given a proper hand over to the colleague covering your duties and to other members of the team, seniors or otherwise? Have you reminded your team you will not be around next week or do you expect them to find out on the day?
- If you are off to teaching but the lecturer does not turn up, will you see an opportunity for a day off, or will you return to your team's duties? If your teaching does not start until late morning, will you see it as an excuse for a lie in, or will you attend the early morning trauma meeting?
- Support other team members. If it is quiet in the ward and you finished your duties early, would you spend the rest of the day in the coffee shop, or will you go down to clinic to ask if an extra hand is needed?
- Be reliable. You may be asked to do a thyroid screen, arrange an urgent doppler, seek a respiratory opinion, contact the plastics in the nearby hospital, arrange a social services referral. If asked to carry out a task, do so, and then inform the rest of the team of its completion. Do not wait for colleagues to come to you, asking again and again as whether the task has been carried out or not. The thyroid tests may take days to complete, the radiologist may be refusing a doppler, the respiratory team may be too busy to attend, the plastics may be in the middle of operating, the social services may need more time to plan a discharge. Even if the task cannot be completed, it is important to let the rest of your colleagues know of the difficulties encountered, and inform them that you are working on it.
- Be punctual, turn up on time. Do not keep wandering around, with the rest of the team looking for you. If you are supposed to be in clinic but you first have to attend the ward, inform your colleagues of this. If you are based in a community practise but an urgent home visit turns up, inform the team of your whereabouts.
- Be flexible and helpful to your colleagues. Professional life is often about give and take. A colleague may ask you to hold their pager whilst they take their son to school, cover their on call at short notice. Try and be accommodative if you can.

- Pay attention to detail, even in small tasks. You may have to gain the trust of others and prove yourself on the small jobs, before you are assigned more complex or more challenging tasks.
- Know the roles of the other team members, know your own role.
- Communicate clearly with the rest of the team (refer to communication chapter).
- Follow the hierarchy of your team as it is vital to ensure adequate team communication, to ensure that all are on board. However, get to know when to go straight to the top.
- Let it be known what you do. As doctors we may often be reluctant to state what we do, fearful to sound as blowing our own trumpet. Unless you inform your seniors of what you get up to, they will not be able to appreciate your hard work. Just because all is running smoothly, it does not mean that everyone is laid back and relaxed. Let it be known how you managed to get that urgent MRI scan, how you taught the medical students to stitch the wound or take bloods, how you coped with all those patients that turned up to your clinic, how you dealt with the run of referrals from the Emergency Department, how difficult it was to go through the microfilmed records and extract the data for your research project. Stating what you do, can help the rest of the team appreciate the need of resources, can help a team justify its role and existence.

Respect the Job

Nothing is a waste of time if you use the experience wisely

Auguste Rodin [4]

At some point in your career, you may end up doing a post which you are not very keen at. You may have to spend time in endocrinology until your respiratory training program starts. You may have to do orthopaedics as part of your general practice rotation. You may want to become a brain surgeon but you end up in psychiatry during your pre-registration years.

The post may not have been your first choice, it may not have been your choice at all. Respect the job, and give it your best self. You are responsible to the patients you are assigned to look after, to the team you are working with. After all, you get paid for doing the job.

If you put the effort, you may gain from each post, no matter how irrelevant to your future you feel that post is. An aspiring physician may gain medical experience looking after unwell patients in an orthopaedic ward. An aspiring Emergency Department doctor may gain suturing experience in gynaecology. An aspiring anaesthetist may learn arterial and central line cannulation in cardiothoracics.

But even if there is no direct clinical gain, learning to give the most, out of respect to the job, is itself a gain. It shows professionalism and good character, which should be recognised and appreciated by seniors and colleagues alike. If you show you are not interested and not put the work into the post, it will be obvious to all those around.

Bring Answers Not Questions

Each problem that I solved became a rule which served afterwards to solve other problems

Rene Descartes [4]

It is easy to come up with a problem or question, and ask someone else for an answer. After all, in medical school, we often learn to look for the answer from a book, our lecturers, or teachers. However, when faced with a problem, rather than formulating a question, try and work out an answer. If there was no one around, what would I do? If left by myself to solve this problem, what would my approach be? When you take a question to a senior or otherwise, think it through, try to come up with an answer or suggestion. In this way, you are not just asking but also offering a solution.

- You see a patient in clinic, take and present a clinical history. You could stop and ask your senior what to do next. Alternatively you could try to formulate a diagnosis, suggest a management plan, suggest how you would investigate the patient further or what treatment to initiate. Even if your thought process or suggestions are incorrect, you would have learnt from the experience, and your effort will be appreciated.
- You have a patient in the ward ready for discharge but you are struggling with home arrangements. Liaise with physiotherapists, social services, occupational therapists, for a workable solution, and present that, rather than throwing the challenge on someone else's desk.

Medicine, but also professional life, is about problem solving. Get into that mindset early on. It is important to show that you put effort into solving the issue, you thought about it and put work into it, rather than simply asking to be spoon fed. The answer does not matter, right or wrong, as long as you can put forwards a logical argument to support it.

You may be in the receiving end, and your juniors or colleagues ask for advice. Encourage them to come up with potential answers, rather than simply questions. You may enjoy solving problems, giving answers, showing what you have gained from years of hard work, learning and experience. However, empower others to think for themselves, to try and work out a feasible solution, rather than simply dictating them an action plan.

It Is Ok to Say "I Do Not Know"

To be persuasive we must be believable; to be believable we must be credible; to be credible we must be truthful

Edward Murrow [12]

If you do not know, it is better to say "I do not know" rather than guessing.

- You took a clinical history and you are presenting it. If questioned about a certain detail you omitted asking the patient about, just say so. It is understandable to omit some information, in a busy clinic, a busy on call.
- You may be asked about the blood results of a patient in the ward, the tests of a patient you admitted. If you forgot to request them or to check if they are back, say so.
- If asked how the ward patients are doing but you have not yet been in the ward that morning, say so.
- If asked a question in an interview for which you do not know the answer, say so, or ask for more information to help you formulate an answer.
- If you can not name the wrist bones, say so, rather than making up names which do not exist.

You can not be expected to know everything, or have an opinion about all issues. No one is expected to have all the answers, not even doctors, and for some questions there may be no answer. Admit what you do not know. If you offer information you did not collect, and you are caught out, your word and credibility may be on the line. Once credibility is gone for such important matters, it is very difficult to regain. It may sound acceptable to make an educated guess in an exam, to guess the most likely correct answer in a multiple choice question, but it is not acceptable to do this in your clinical, or professional practise. Be accurate and truthful, about the information you give, to gain the confidence and trust of others.

Understand Your Limitations

If you accept your limitations you go beyond them

Brendan Francis [4]

Act within your abilities and be safe. It is often a fine balance between ensuring you act within your limits but avoiding looking non confident, not knowledgeable, looking as if you are responsibility shy. Know the limitations of your knowledge, clinical abilities, persuasive abilities, authority, expertise.

- If a clinical problem or procedure is beyond your skills, ask for help or refer it on.
- If you reach a dead end in trying to make a diagnosis, ask for another opinion. A fresh pair of eyes may help see things in new brighter light.
- Your position may not allow you to successfully refer a patient on or obtain a radiological investigation. Escalate to your seniors, whose word may carry more weight.
- You may be asked to give an expert opinion about the prospects of returning to work following an injury. Are you really able to assess that? Would an occupational specialist be better equipped to do so?

Know when to escalate and know whom to escalate to. You will not be criticised for asking for advice or help, but could be susceptible to criticism if you do not ask and things go wrong.

You may be the first on call at hospital and your more seniors are on call from home. It maybe late at night and your seniors may be asleep. If you need to ask, do so. A common concern is that, if on call, for which cases should you inform your senior? This will depend on your seniority, your capabilities, your specialty, your local arrangements. Some situations to consider are:

- For an unwell patient the management of who requires a senior's skills or knowledge.
- For controversial issues, to discuss the best line of action.
- If a high profile person gets admitted; better for your senior to find out from you, rather than from the newspapers the next morning.

Ask Questions

The art and science of asking questions is the source of all knowledge
Thomas Berger [4]

No matter how simple the question may sound, no matter how obvious the answer may look, if in doubt ask. Very likely, your trainers or seniors were in your shoes at some point, even if they seem reluctant to admit it. Asking often means learning, and it is important to learn the basics at an early stage, before you move up.

- You may see a patient with a finger tip open fracture. Do you wash it in the Emergency Department or do you take them to theatre for that? If taking them to theatre when do you do so? In the middle of the night? The next day?
- Someone may be having a heart attack. Do you start them on aspirin? If so how much?
- The radiograph is reported as showing a pneumothorax. How do you distinguish that from the surrounding air in the lungs?
- Someone presents with a large boil. Do you give antibiotics or do you slash it open?

Ask and ask again. No matter how basic the question seems, no matter how obvious the answer may be. Even if it is just to confirm that you are right, ask if you need to. Ask different people. You may ask several trainers to clarify the same issue. Different people may be able to explain things in different ways, ask more than one if needed. If in a lecture or group teaching, you may feel embarrassed to ask; what will the teacher think, what will your peers think? If there is an area that you do not understand, there is a good chance a substantial proportion of the audience does not understand that either but are too worried to ask.

Avoid Cutting Corners

Never cut corners, or accept anything that's second-rate

Bruce Oldfield [4]

We live in a fast world where rapid answers and actions are demanded. There are time pressures, workload pressures, financial constraints.

If you feel that you need to further investigate a medical problem, do so. If you feel that you need specialist equipment for operating, demand that is available. Be safe, stick to the book, and you will be respected for it. The main aim is to cause no harm, to give the best of your ability.

In August 2001, Air Transat Flight 236 flying from Toronto to Lisbon, suffered complete power loss over the Atlantic Ocean due to its fuel running out. Its experienced pilots managed to glide and safely land the plane in Azores. The Airbus A330 run out of fuel due to an engine fuel leak caused by an incorrect part installed in its hydraulics system. Subsequent investigation reported several factors accounting for this catastrophic failure. However, it was of note that during the engine change, the lead technician relied on verbal advice rather than acquiring access to the relevant engine service bulletin, a practise considered essential for proper engine installation. Time-pressures to complete the work in time for a scheduled flight, and to clear the hangar for another use, were quoted as factors that may have influenced the reliance simply on verbal advice [14].

If you do not feel at your best, then HALT [15]. This acronym, used to warn those recovering from addictions as to when they are more vulnerable to relapse, may also be used in the workplace. If you are:

H-ungry
A-ngry
L-ate
or **T**-ired,

take a pause, take a deep breath, take a step back. Avoid rushed decisions, rushed actions, avoid cutting corners.

Have a Plan B and a Plan C

If plan A doesn't work, the alphabet has 25 more letters – 204 if you're in Japan
                                                                        Claire Cook [12]

Have a plan as how to do things your preferred way but have alternative plans, if things do not work out. Have a back up plan. Follow your preferred route but be prepared to take another road if you get stuck.

- You may be getting blood for a blood screen. What if you can not get any veins?
- You may be fixing a hip fracture. What if the fracture is too shattered and can not be fixed?
- You may be taking an appendix out through a laparoscope. What if the appendix has burst?
- What if you drop your saw on the floor in the middle of knee surgery? Do you have another on the shelf?
- You may set up a randomised trial. What if recruitment rate is poor at 6 months?
- You are sitting your fellowship exams. What if unsuccessful?
- Going for a new post interview. What if you do not get it?
- You may be treating someone with asthma. What if inhalers are not good enough?
- You may be taking a child to theatre with a pulseless hand for fracture reduction. What if the pulses do not return after you put the bones back? Should you warn the vascular team well in advance?

A football coach may bring on substitutes if the team is not playing hard, a parachutist has a backup chute, a pilot may log in a divergent route; should you not have an alternative plan? Try to predict the potential difficulties you may face for your day to day tasks. Plan how to deal with these before they arise. Have, not just one, but multiple alternate plans. To be prepared is professional, having alternate plans is a measure of good judgement.

Strive for Excellence

Perfection is not attainable, but if we chase perfection we can catch excellence

Vince Lombardi [4]

Strive for continuous improvement. Aim high, aim for the best possible, in what ever discipline you find yourself in, whatever tasks you undertake. Aim for the best achievable, whether these are clinical skills, technical skills, teaching skills, managerial tasks, or research activities. The best achievable may vary according to the system you are practising in, your support and resources. Consider the following:

- Train to the best standards – both for clinical and non-clinical skills.
- Learn from the best – the best may be on the other side of the world, or may simply be next door, in your institution or department.
- Adopt successful systems and policies – learn from successful, well functioning institutions. How did they achieve that? What are their systems and structures? How can you adopt their success to your practise? Why start from scratch if others have already led the way?
- Keep up with current evidence – long lasting questions are continuously getting answered. Controversies and queries are resolved. Keep up to date with an evolving medical world. Use the best evidence in your day to day practise.

Set high standards for practise, aim for continuous improvement, and try your best to achieve those.

Seek and Give Feedback

Feedback is the breakfast of champions

Ken Blanchard [4]

Feedback is paramount in professional development. Your personal perceptions for your performance may differ from the views of others. Ask for constructive feedback for what you do. Ask for feedback with regards your clinical skills, communication skills, professionalism, managerial or teaching skills.

Feedback may be verbal or written. It may be formal or informal. Seek feedback from your seniors, juniors, peers. Seek feedback from patients, other doctors and non-medical staff. Seek feedback not only from those you expect favourable views, but also from those who may criticise you. Listen to feedback and address any areas for further improvement.

In giving feedback be honest and frank, but try and be constructive. Praise the positives, highlight what went well, whilst also acknowledging what could be improved, what could have been done better. Giving feedback may fill you with authority, you may be eager to express your opinion. However, consider giving the individual concerned the chance to judge their own performance, in a critical way, before you rush to say what you think.

You may be asked by a junior to assess their clinical examination skills, history taking, surgical performance, presentation in the departmental teaching. You may be asked by a peer for feedback as how they managed the last departmental meeting, how they handled a difficult situation, how they dealt with a difficult colleague.

An approach of giving feedback is the following:

- Ask the individual

  - "What do you think went really well?"
  - "Is there anything you would do differently next time?"

- State your evaluation of the performance

  - Start by pointing out the good things.
  - State what could have been done better.

Keep an Open Mind for Change

To improve is to change; to be perfect is to change often

Winston Churchill [4]

We live in a fast world. Standards are rising, the public is becoming more demanding, redundant practises are scrutinised. The aim is not only to provide high quality safe medical care, but also provide care that is cost effective, and easily accessible. Technology is advancing rapidly and the medical workplace can not stay immune from such advances. Keep an open mind for new ways of working, for new applications of technology.

It maybe that printed radiographs are to be replaced with electronic equivalents. It maybe that traditional letter dictating and typing is to be replaced by voice recognition systems. It maybe that medical records move from a written to an electronic format. It maybe that requests or referrals have to be sent via email rather than through the post. It maybe consultations are to be done over the phone to reduce unnecessary hospital attendances. It maybe that out of hours working gives patients easier access to clinics. It maybe that outcome results will be audited through a national database. It maybe that new anaesthetic techniques can reduce post-surgery hospital stay. It maybe that braces and splints can be custom made with three dimensional printing. It maybe that technically challenging surgery can be performed more safely with computer guided or robotic assistance.

Keep an open mind in facing potential change, rather than dismissing it at first glance. The process of change may be challenging, but its outcome may well worth it. Engage in the change process, as that may help you shape the new order. As a frontline doctor you are in a unique position to facilitate that, since you know first hand what your patients are asking for, and what the challenges of the workplace are. Whatever your seniority, you may make a positive contribution, showing that you have the common interest at heart, as an integral team member. Give constructive suggestions that will help ensure changes are workable, applicable, and effective. If you distance your self, you may stand by as a mere observer. Most likely, change will still happen.

Respect the Resources

Too many people spend money they haven't earned, to buy things they don't want, to impress people they don't like

Will Rogers [4]

Costs of healthcare are rising. Life expectancy is increasing. New, more costly treatments are becoming available. Pressures on healthcare systems are mounting. In the USA, costs of health care rose from $253 billion in 1980 to $2.6 trillion in 2010. Up to $700 billion of this, could be eliminated, without compromising quality of care [16–20].

Whatever your role in healthcare provision, whatever stage of career you are, respect the resources available. Question expenses, identify areas of wastage, propose and implement cost efficient care. Lower cost does not necessarily mean lower quality care. The skill is to distinguish between cost reducing, but quality maintaining measures, and cost reducing measures which may impair clinical care.

Simple ideas can result in massive savings. Should you be opening disposables unless you definitely need them? Should you not be turning off the lights and computer after you finished? Could some equipment you are about to throw away, be recycled and used again? If it were your own money would you be spending it differently?

Question the cost of new medicines, the cost of new implants. A survey of 503 Orthopaedic surgeons in the USA, showed that participants were able to estimate the cost of implants they used, only about 20 % of time [21]. Medicines and implants are produced by an industry which invests in them, and is looking at making a profit. Many of these companies are on the stock market, and are accountable to shareholders. Representatives of such companies may visit you to try and promote their products.

Much of the money industry spends is on marketing rather than the development of new products. It was estimated that in 2004, the pharmaceutical marketing expenditures in the USA mounted at $57.5 billion as compared to $31.5 billion for research and development [22].

A lot of new developments may be industry driven, as old patents are running out. New treatments many not necessarily improve outcomes. Question the cost of new products and new developments, rather than taking them for granted, seek evidence to support their effectiveness and superiority over traditional treatments.

Stick to the Rules

> You have to learn the rules of the game. And then you have to play better than anyone else
>
> Albert Einstein [4]

Follow the regulations and rules of your employer, your team, your department, your institution, your training program, your regulatory body.

You may not agree with some of these rules, you may feel they do not make sense, that they are counter-productive, short sighted, and unfair. You may be opposing the rule of having to give 6 weeks notice before you can go on holidays, that not all juniors can be away at the same time, and that you can not transfer holiday days from one attachment to the next. You may not agree with the rules of having to do countless work based assessments, or having to get published in order to complete your training.

If so, express your opinion, campaign to change those rules, but follow them in the meantime. Rules may at sometimes look lax or loosely applied. However, if rules are clearly laid out and you decide to go your own way, you may leave yourself open to criticism and be held to account.

If the circumstances demand to seek an exemption, follow the appropriate routes to put your case forwards, well in advance, and ask for such lineage. Breaking the rules with retrospective explanations, may simply look as coming up with excuses.

If unsure what the rules are, seek clarification, and follow them to the line. For any system or organisation to function, in a cohesive way, the rules ought to be respected and obeyed.

Dress Appropriately

Whether it's because of how somebody looks or because of what they're wearing, you kind of assess a person in the first five minutes before they even speak

Shemar Moore [4]

How we dress, how we look, may influence how we are viewed, both by patients and other staff, with regards to our authority and credibility. How we dress may also reflect how we perceive and respect our working environment, the organisation we work in, our colleagues and patients. How you decide to dress may depend on personal and cultural preferences, which part of the world you practice in, your exact duties, whether you are based in wards or clinics.

There are no hard rules as how to dress, but consider:

- Follow the guidance of your employer, if one exists. There may be a requirement for a uniform, a ban on ties and long sleeves (as a policy of infection control, despite the lack of sound scientific evidence behind it [23, 24]), a ban on jewellery and makeup.
- Dress comfortably to facilitate your daily duties. You may cover wards throughout the hospital, you may be on the crash call, are high heels really the best choice? You may look good in tight trousers, but should you worry about the buttons bursting undone, every time you kneel to take bloods?
- Be guided by your patients. If your patients dress smartly to visit you in clinic, would it be appropriate for you to turn up in jeans, T-shirts and flip-flops?
- Be guided by the rest of the team. If all seniors turn up in shirt and trousers, how would the most junior look turning up in black suit and bow tie?

Sotgiu et al. [25] surveyed 765 Italian medical and surgical patients. Most preferred doctors wearing formal attire with a white coat. Casual or semi-formal attire were the least preferred. Respondents felt that it was inappropriate for doctors to have long hair, visible tattoos, body piercing, or excessive makeup. Rehman et al. [26] evaluated 400 patients and visitors at a medical outpatients clinic, in the USA. Seventy six percent favoured professional attire with white coat, followed by surgical scrubs, business and then casual dress. Their trust and confidence with the doctors correlated with their preference for professional attire. Respondents reported that they would be more willing to share personal issues such as social, sexual or psychological problems with a doctor who is professionally dressed. Aitken et al. [27] evaluated patients and relatives views in an orthopaedic outpatients clinic. The most popular preference for doctors' attire was smart casual clothing. Patients reported that cleanliness and good personal hygiene may be more important than clothing style.

If still in doubt dress smartly, look tidy and respectable, blend in with the crowd.

Use Social Network Sites Wisely

Social media is changing the way we communicate and the way we are perceived, both positively and negatively. Every time you post a photo, or update your status, you are contributing to your own digital footprint and personal brand

Amy Jo Martin [4]

Recent years have seen an explosion of social network sites. Face book, Twitter, LinkedIn, YouTube, and Blogger are only some of those to mention. Facebook has about 1.32 billion active users, of whom 829 million are daily users [28]. Profiles may be accessed by anyone, especially if privacy settings are not applied. Even when such settings are applied, a profile may still be accessed by friends of friends, estimated for an average USA user at 45,000 other users [29].

Social media allows you to keep in touch with friends and family, sharing moments, news, and events, but can also provide beneficial healthcare uses. They allow discussions between professionals with regards healthcare, research and front-line developments, sharing of information with regards upcoming educational events. At the same time, social media provide an easy access to the public with regards information about medical conditions. Social media may also provide easy access to information about medical professionals, their clinical interests and expertise.

However, when it comes to doctors, social media may carry some challenges [30–35]. Moments of lapse may allow postings that could adversely affect how the individual doctor is viewed, or how the medical profession is perceived. Comments may be taken out of context and give unintended impressions. Once information is out in the public it may be very difficult, if not impossible, to retract. Rocha and de Castro [36] examined the frequency with which students from a Brazilian medical school came across unprofessional online behaviour of other medical students or physicians. 13.7 % of participants reported witnessing acts of violating patient's privacy, whilst 85.4 % reported witnessing photos showing consumption of alcohol. Clyde et al. [29] evaluated the impressions of professionalism given by different face book profiles of medical doctors in the USA. Profiles that contained healthy behaviours (such as reading or hiking) were rated as the most professional. Unhealthy profiles (picturing behaviours such as overeating or sleeping in) were rated as the least professional.

Recently, several professional or regulatory medical bodies, have produced guidance with regards social medial use [37, 38]. In using social media consider the following:

- Avoid posting unprofessional material – offensive jokes, self embarrassment photos, unhealthy activities.
- Avoid posting confidential information about patients, colleagues, workplace.
- Ensure that any security settings, limiting who can access the posted information, are set on.
- Keep patient doctor boundaries clear.

Social network sites are essentially another form of public communication. Treat it as you would treat any other means, with the professionalism they deserve. Freedom of expression applies to the web for all individuals, medical and non-medical professionals alike. However, as in verbal communication, it is not only what is said that matters, but also how it is said, and how it is perceived.

References

1. Royal College of Physicians of London (RCPL). Doctors in society: medical professionalism in a changing world. London: RCPL; 2005.
2. Stern DT. A framework for measuring professionalism. In: Dt S, editor. Measuring medical professionalism. New York: Oxford University Press; 2006.
3. Wilkinson TJ, Wade WB, Knock LD. A blueprint to assess professionalism: results of a systematic review. Acad Med. 2009;84(5):551–8.
4. Famous quotes at brainy quote. www.brainyquote.com. Accessed on 23 Sept 2014.
5. Darzi A. Undercover surgeon: the night porter chronicle. BMJ. 2013;347:f7277.
6. Back K, Back K. Assertiveness at work: a practical guide to handling awkward situations. 3rd ed. London: McGraw-Hill Publishing Company; 2005.
7. Williams C. Overcoming depression and low mood. A five areas approach. 3rd ed. London,UK: Hodder Arnold; 2012.
8. Garelick A, Fagin L. Doctor to doctor: getting on with colleagues. Adv Psychiatr Treat. 2004;10:225–32.
9. Faruqui RA, Ikkos G. Poorly performing supervisors and trainers of trainee doctors. Psychiatr Bull. 2007;31:148–52.
10. Oxford dictionaries. www.oxforddictionaries.com. Accessed on 23 Sept 2014.
11. Living language. http://www.livinglanguage.com. Accessed on 25 Sept 2014.
12. Goodreads. http://www.goodreads.com. Accessed on 25 Sept 2014.
13. Vince lombardi quotes. http://www.vincelombardi.com. Accessed on 25 Sept 2014.
14. All engines-out landing due to fuel exhaustion. 2001. http://www.fss.aero/accident-reports. Accessed on 25 Sept 2014.
15. Zomerland G. H.A.L.T.: a self care tool. http://www.chinnstreetcounseling.com. Accessed on 25 Sept 2014.
16. Logio L, Dine CJ, Smith CD. High-value, cost conscious care: Less is more. Acad Intern Med Insight. 2013;11(1):16–7.
17. Cooke M. Cost consciousness in patient care–what is medical education's responsibility? N Engl J Med. 2010;362(14):1253–5.
18. Weinberger SE. Providing high-value, cost-conscious care: a critical 7th general competency for physicians. Ann Intern Med. 2011;155:386–8.
19. Nand B. Doctors should be taught to consider the cost of their practice. BMJ. 2014;348:g2629.
20. Brody H. Medicine's ethical responsibility for health care reform: the top five list. N Engl J Med. 2010;362:283–5.
21. Okike K, O'Toole RV, Pollak AN, Bishop JA, McAndrew CM, Mehta S, Cross 3rd WW, Garrigues GE, Harris MB, Lebrun CT. Survey finds few orthopedic surgeons know the costs of the devices they implant. Health Aff (Millwood). 2014;33(1):103–9.
22. Gagnon MA, Lexchin J. The cost of pushing pills: a new estimate of pharmaceutical promotion expenditures in the United States. PLoS Med. 2008;5(1):e1.
23. Burger A, Wijewardena C, Clayson S, Greatorex RA. Bare below elbows: does this policy affect handwashing efficacy and reduce bacterial colonisation? Ann R Coll Surg Engl. 2011;93(1):13–6.
24. Willis-Owen CA, Subramanian P, Kumari P, Houlihan-Burne D. Effects of 'bare below the 'elbows' policy on hand contamination of 92 hospital doctors in a district general hospital. J Hosp Infect. 2010;75(2):116–9.
25. Sotgiu G, Nieddu P, Mameli L, Sorrentino E, Pirina P, Porcu A, Madeddu S, Idini M, Di Martino M, Delitala G, Mura I, Dore MP. Evidence for preferences of Italian patients for physician attire. Patient Prefer Adherence. 2012;6:361–7.
26. Rehman SU, Nietert PJ, Cope DW, Kilpatrick AO. What to wear to-day? Effect of doctor's attire on the trust and confidence of patients. Am J Med. 2005;118(11):1279–86.
27. Aitken SA, Tinning CG, Gupta S, Medlock G, Wood AM, Aitken MA. The importance of the orthopaedic doctors' appearance: a cross-regional questionnaire based study. Surgeon. 2014;12(1):40–6.
28. Facebook newsroom. http://newsroom.fb.com/company-info/. 17 Aug.

29. Clyde JW, Domenech Rodríguez MM, Geiser C. Medical professionalism: an experimental look at physicians' facebook profiles. Med Educ Online. 2014;19:23149.
30. DeCamp M, Cunningham AM. Social media: the way forward or a waste of time for physicians? J R Coll Physicians Edinb. 2013;43(4):318–22.
31. DeCamp M, Koenig TW, Chisolm MS. Social media and physicians' online identity crisis. JAMA. 2013;310(6):581–2.
32. Greysen SR, Kind T, Chretien KC. Online professionalism and the mirror of social media. J Gen Intern Med. 2010;25(11):1227–9.
33. Gholami-Kordkheili F, Wild V, Strech D. The impact of social media on medical professionalism: a systematic qualitative review of challenges and opportunities. J Med Internet Res. 2013;15(8):e184.
34. Azu MC, Lilley EJ, Kolli AH. Social media, surgeons, and the internet: an era or an error? Am Surg. 2012;78(5):555–8.
35. Ross S, Lai K, Walton JM, Kirwan P, White JS. "I have the right to a private life": medical students' views about professionalism in a digital world. Med Teach. 2013;35(10):826–31.
36. Rocha PN, de Castro NA. Opinions of students from a Brazilian medical school regarding online professionalism. J Gen Intern Med. 2014;29(5):758–64.
37. Doctors' use of social media. 2013. http://www.gmc-uk.org/guidance/ethical_guidance. Accessed 27 Sept 2014.
38. Farnan JM, Snyder Sulmasy L, Worster BK, Chaudhry HJ, Rhyne JA, Arora VM, American College of Physicians Ethics, Professionalism and Human Rights Committee, American College of Physicians Council of Associates, Federation of State Medical Boards Special Committee on Ethics and Professionalism. Online medical professionalism: patient and public relationships: policy statement from the American College of Physicians and the Federation of State Medical Boards. Ann Intern Med. 2013;158(8):620–7.

Chapter 5
Learning and Teaching

A doctor's life is often one of continuous learning. With the progress of Medicine it is important to stay up to date with developments and advancements. New roles with career progression means that further knowledge has to be acquired, new skills (clinical or non-clinical) to be mastered.

As doctors we learn from didactical teaching, whereby we are told or shown how to do things. We learn from discussions with colleagues and peers, through doing, and through teaching those around us. Each of these methods has its place and merits in the long journey of continuous learning.

Similarly, as doctors we aim to disseminate knowledge or pass on skills. We may thus find ourselves teaching other healthcare practitioners, medical students, junior doctors, peers or senior colleagues.

This chapter examines the various learning methods. Advice is given as how to make the most of each learning opportunity, and how to deliver well constructed, successful teaching. Advice is also given about preparing for post-graduate exams, assessing trainees, and organising medical courses.

© Springer International Publishing Switzerland 2015
C. Panayiotou Charalambous, *Career Skills for Doctors*,
DOI 10.1007/978-3-319-13479-6_5

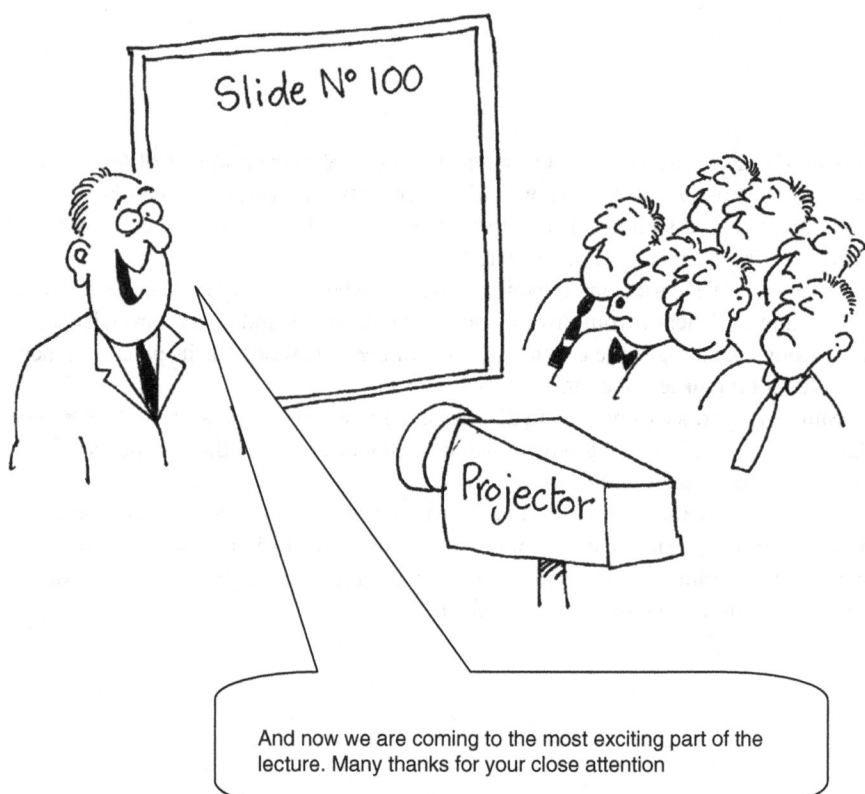

Principles of Learning and Teaching

Tell me and I forget. Teach me and I remember. Involve me and I learn
Benjamin Franklin [1]

In learning and teaching consider the following principles:

- Individuals may have different learning preferences, that is particular ways of learning.
- Previous knowledge and experience can act as the platform for acquiring new knowledge.
- Different teaching methods exist, both active and passive.
- Learning and retention of new knowledge may be influenced by the teaching methods employed.
- There is a learning curve in acquiring a new skill.

Learning Preferences

Educationalists Rita and Kenneth Dunn proposed that a number of factors may influence the ability to learn [2, 3]. These factors may be environmental (environment of learning), sociological (whom we learn with), emotional (attitude to learning), physiological (how we engage with learning) and psychological (how information is processed). In considering physiological factors, learners may be described as:

1. Visual – preference for learning through seeing – pictures, charts, graphs, illustrations.
2. Auditory – preference for learning through listening – lectures, tapes, listening to someone explaining it, listening to own self repeating it.
3. Kinaesthetic or tactile – preference for learning through handling things, touching and feeling – practical workshops.

Not all factors are important for all individuals, and each learner may have a unique combination of preferences. You may recognise what type of learner you mainly are. Appreciating what type of learner you are is important, in trying to reach out for those learning tools and methods, that will allow you to maximise your learning efficiency, and hence play at your strengths.

When teaching, understanding your learners preferences could enable you to individualise the teaching methods you employ. However, if dealing with a large group of students, such an individual approach may be difficult. Nevertheless, by incorporating teaching methods which provide for several learning styles, you may influence more of your learners.

Experiential Learning

The value of experience is not in seeing much, but in seeing wisely

William Osler [1]

David Kolb, an American educationalist, believes that "learning is a process whereby knowledge is created through the transformation of experience" [4]. In the theory of experiential learning, Kolb described a four stage model of learning (Fig. 5.1). In the initial stage, we experience a learning event, and in the second stage we reflect on what took place and what we observed. In the third stage, we try to analyse and come up with a model as to what we learnt, whereas in the final stage, one plans how to act in the future based on the model or theory developed. This can then be applied in practise, leading to further encounters and experiences.

In Medicine, we often refer to the importance of gaining experience. We aim for gaining experience through volume, encounter of unusual cases, repetition of tasks, observations of events. Yet, as Kolb's cycle suggests, experience is not a passive process, one to be assimilated simply by our mere presence, but is an active process, requiring input and reflection on the learner's part.

The theory of experiential learning also suggests that learning is effective when based on previous experience. In trying to work out as what to do in a new situation, one can look back at previous experiences as a guide of further action. Principles acquired through participation in one event may help one to work out a solution, when faced with a new problem. Aim to learn principles and concepts that may allow you to work out the answer to a question or the solution to a problem, rather than simply trying to memorise and recall detailed facts.

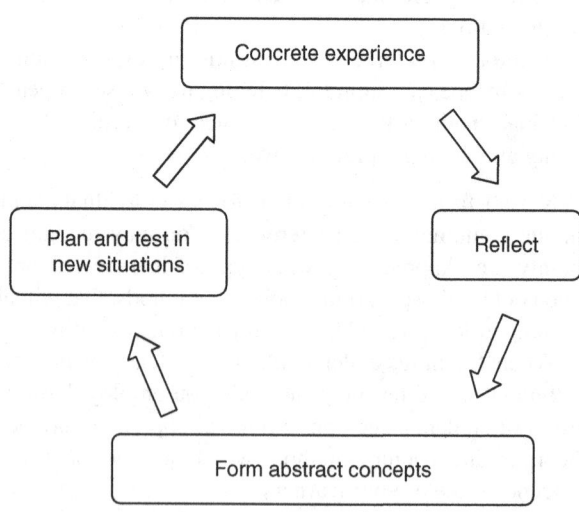

Fig. 5.1 Kolb's cycle of learning (Adapted from Kolb [4])

Learning Styles

Learning may be either passive or active. In passive learning, the learner acts as the mere receiver of transmitted information, whilst in active learning, the learner is a participating player. Three commonly used approaches for teaching, and hence learning, are the didactic, Socratic, and facilitative [5]:

- Didactic – passing on of information or facts, with very little participation on the learner's part.
- Socratic – mastered by the Greek philosopher Socrates, it describes a method whereby the teacher uses a step by step questioning, to help lead the learner towards the solution to a problem.
- Facilitative – the learners per se take an active role, in deciding as to what to be learnt, and the learning approaches to be used. The teacher facilitates, helps, and supports this learning environment. Problem based learning is increasingly used in medical education. Learners are given a clinical or other scenario based on which they identify areas to explore and set their learning objectives. Learners look for the information that will allow them to meet these objectives, and then meet and discuss this information as a way of learning. A facilitator may ensure that learners cover all expected areas, according to syllabus or curriculum, and do not deviate from what the scenario aims to achieve.

At different times you may use one or a combination of these learning styles, both when you are yourself learning, or as a teacher in trying to engage your students.

Pyramid of Learning

The Pyramid of Learning (Fig. 5.2), describes how the degree of retention varies according to the way we receive information (teaching methods). According to this, we remember 5 % of information gained from lectures, 10 % of what we read, 20 %

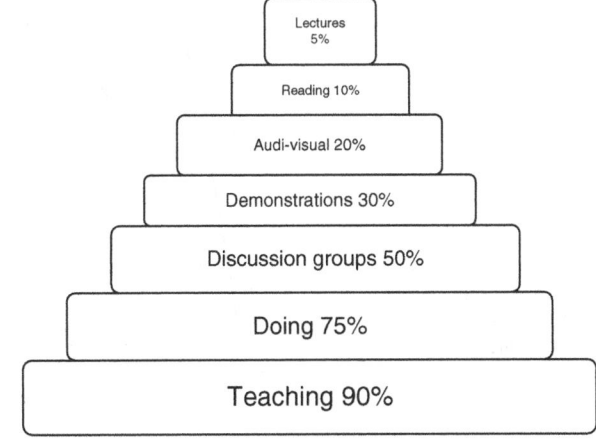

Fig. 5.2 Learning Pyramid – learning methods and retention rates (Adapted from Masters [6])

of information presented with audio-visual means, 30 % of what we see and hear in demonstrations, 50 % by participating in discussions, 75 % of what we do, and 90 % of what we teach [6].

The Pyramid of Learning is attributed to research by the National Training Laboratories for Applied Behavioural Sciences, USA, but with no published data to support the proposed proportions [7]. Even though the origin of the Pyramid and the actual proportions have been questioned, it demonstrates that the more actively we engage in learning, the more likely it is to retain new knowledge and information. Doing and teaching allows us to engage deeply with a learning event and hence retain knowledge better, than when simply spoon fed with information.

Recognising the Learning Curve

Most skills, clinical, technical, or otherwise, have a learning curve. This curve essentially describes how performance varies with time, and with the accumulation of more and more experience.

A steep curve means that fast learning can be achieved over a short period of time, whilst a shallower curve requires more time to reach a plateau of effective performance (Fig. 5.3). It is important to recognise the relationship between the slope of the learning curve and the complexity of the skill to be mastered. It is a misnomer to refer to complex activities as ones that have a steep curve, as it is the difficult tasks that may take more time to acquire and hence have a more gradual

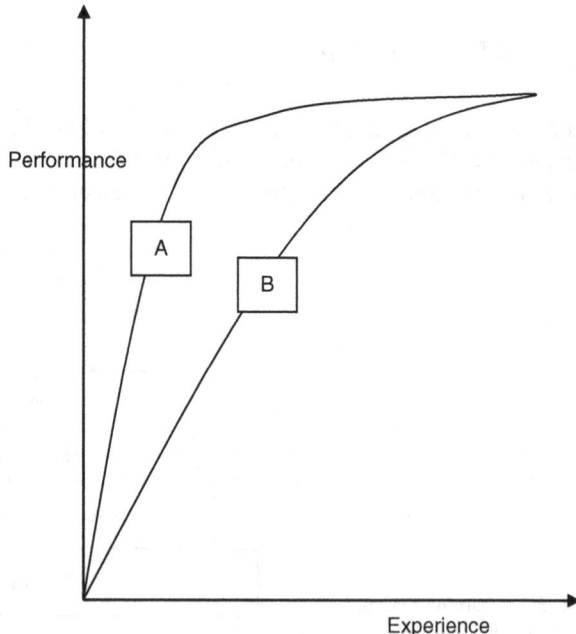

Fig. 5.3 Learning curve. Skill A has a steeper curve, but is acquired much faster than skill B

ascend. Easy tasks may be learnt more quickly, hence, giving a quick, steep rise, to skilful practise.

In acquiring a new skill it is important to recognise this curve. Be realistic as to how hard a skill is, and how much time is needed to acquire a new skill. When things do not go smoothly, appreciate that you may still be on your learning curve, and there is still potential for further learning. Appreciate that whilst ascending the curve, support from peers, colleagues or seniors may be needed.

Learning from Teaching Events

Certain behaviours may help you improve your learning experiences through different means of teaching (didactic, Socratic, facilitative) and also in different settings (lectures, courses, workshops, large group, small group, one to one teaching):

- Choose courses and other educational events wisely. Examine their contents, seek advice from colleagues or seniors as whether they are worth attending.
- Choose teaching events that will provide knowledge you can soon apply in practise, and can enhance your day to day performance.

    - If doing an endocrinology post in a medical rotation, attending a thyroid symposium may be of greater value than attending a heart auscultation course.
    - If doing a knee surgery post, attending an arthroscopic knee course may help you follow arthroscopic procedures or improve your day to day surgical skills, and be more relevant than attending a hand course.

- Do pre-course reading. Go prepared to get the most out of it. View the event almost like a revision, rather than initial learning. Have queries you need clarifying, questions you need answered. It may be a unique opportunity to meet and directly question the originator of a concept or other experts in a particular field.
- Revise what you learnt shortly after the event, when all is still fresh and clear in your mind.
- Make notes, either during or after the event, something concrete to refer to at a later stage.
- Learn simple concepts early, get the basics cleared first, before advancing on.
- Learn from colleagues, seniors and juniors alike. Do not concentrate simply on your trainer's professional title, but rather on their knowledge, message and skills.
- Set your learning needs. Make it clear as what you expect from an educational event, and give feedback if not up to standard.
- Enjoy learning. Look at questioning as thought provocation rather than uncomfortable interrogation.

Continuity of Care and Learning

Continuity of care refers to a stable, continuous relationship between patient and doctor. Continuity of care may improve patient satisfaction and enhance communication [8], but is also important in a doctor's learning and training.

Follow patients through. With reduced working hours and shift work, it is becoming more and more difficult to follow the journey of patients through the healthcare system. Yet continuity of care is a vital learning tool. Continuity of care may provide one of the most direct feedbacks you get in clinical practise.

- You admitted a patient with shortness of breath whilst on night shift. When next back at work, enquire as to what happened. Was your diagnosis of heart failure right? Was the treatment you started appropriate?
- You made a diagnosis in clinic and sent the patient for more tests. Did you get it right? What was the outcome of the investigations?
- You assessed a patient but the clinical findings were inconclusive. What did it turn out to be?
- You operated or assisted in an operation. Did surgery help? Did symptoms improve? Any post-operative complications? How did the patient do day by day whilst in hospital? How long did it take for the symptoms to get better?
- You reported the MRI scan of a patient's abdomen who then had surgery. What did the surgeons find, how did it relate to your interpretation of the scan?
- You referred a patient to the Emergency Department. What was the outcome? Could the patient have been managed in the community?
- You excised a skin lesion. Did the histological examination of the lesion confirm your clinical diagnosis?

Learning Through Simulation

The reduction of working hours, legislation fears, and targets for service provision, have reduced, in many settings, the learning opportunities encountered in clinical practise. Simulation refers to the artificial representation of a real life process [9]. Simulation can provide an invaluable tool, in preparing you in how to act when encountering a new situation, in preparing you for the real event, in allowing you to practise and develop your skills.

Pilots do not learn how to deal with in-flight emergencies only when in the cockpit, musicians do not learn how to play instruments only through live concerts, the military do not learn how to fight only when in battle, astronauts do not practise their landing gear only when on the moon. Why should doctors only practise our skills in real life situations?

Simulation may enable you to acquire new, and improve existing skills, whilst moving the learning curve away from the clinical environment, away from the patient. It allows you to make mistakes and learn from them, with no harm occurring. With simulation the "see one, do one approach" [10–15] to learning and experience becomes redundant. Amongst others, simulation may help in developing:

- Technical skills (life-support techniques, cannulation, urinary catheterisation, intubation, surgical procedures).
- Clinical examination skills (chest auscultation, breast, pelvic, rectal examination).
- Clinical management skills.
- Communication skills.
- Crisis management skills (crash call, failure of the anaesthetic machine, plane crash landing in nearby airport with many injured).
- Team working, people management, leadership skills.

Even if you do not have access to expensive high technology simulators, pristine manikins, or shiny simulating centres, you can still make the most of simulation. You may ask the representative of the company providing the bone fracture fixation plates to bring some saw bones to practise fracture plating. A trip to the local butcher may provide specimens to help your chest drain insertion techniques. Constructing and practising a crisis scenario may improve your team building skills.

Make the most of simulation, practise and practise again.

Learning in Training Posts

Learning, regardless of how it is defined, is ultimately the responsibility of the learner, not the teacher

Bob Kizlik [1]

In your training years you may work in formal or informal training posts. In making the most of such training posts, it is important to get to own your training. Set your goals, identify your needs, request the processes that will let you meet those needs. Have an initial, mid-attachment, and end of attachment meeting with your supervisor. Prepare for these and use them effectively.

- Initial meeting

  - Establish who is, or are, facilitating your training.
  - Help your supervisor to establish a clear understanding of your career stage, knowledge level, experience.
  - Identify areas that may have been highlighted in previous attachments, that need to be addressed.
  - Identify what you aim to get out of the post.
  - Explore learning opportunities – attending specialised theatre lists, attending chronic pain clinics.
  - Identify special circumstances, plans for holidays or study leave.
  - Agree to specific targets.
  - Know whom to contact if any difficulties.
  - Set days for middle and final meeting.

- Middle meeting

  - Assess progress
  - If things not progressing as you would expect bring this to your trainer's attention early. Raising such issues at the end of your post may help future trainees, but may not directly help you.
  - Assess achievements and identify further areas of improvement.
  - Contingency plan to meet original targets.

- Final meeting

  - Reflection of how the attachment went.
  - Complete all necessary paperwork on time.
  - Which training targets have you met.
  - What needs to be addressed in your next attachment.

Postgraduate Exams

Examinations are formidable even to the best prepared, for the greatest fool may ask more than the wisest man can answer

Charles Caleb Colton [1]

For many the primary aim at medical school was studying, learning, attending teaching, and passing exams, with some of us having to work on the side to help fund our studies. After graduating these roles often reverse. It is likely that most of you will be working, whilst at the same time having to study as part of continuous professional development, or for preparing and sitting postgraduate exams. Postgraduate exams are often in the form of written papers, demonstration of clinical skills or oral questioning (vivas). Each of these examination types may require different preparation and learning techniques. As the time available for studying is often limited, efficient exam preparation is essential. In preparing for postgraduate exams you may consider:

- Decide well in advance as to when to sit the exams. Factors to take into account are:

  - How well prepared can you be by the exam date?
  - What post will you be doing at that time? Is it likely to be a busy post? Is it going to be a job where you want to get as much clinical experience as possible or a quieter one where you can afford to take more time out for revision?
  - How many times are you allowed to take the exam? If there is no limit is it worth considering sit the exam as a form of practise? If there is a limit on times allowed should you not be sitting it until fully ready? Even with the best preparation exams may not go as planned. Better not sit an exam until there is a good chance of passing. Failing an exam is an uncomfortable experience, and may hinder morale and motivation for further preparation.
  - Give ample time to prepare for the exam. Try and put aside some time every day for revising. Leaving it all for the last 2 weeks might have worked in the medical school, but may not be the best option in postgraduate assessments.

- Passing exams is not just about knowledge but also about technique. Tailor your revision to the exam. Preparing for multiple choice questions, where detailed factual knowledge is essential, is different from preparing for a clinical viva where communication skills, ability to answer with confidence, and ability to give well constructed, structured answers are more important. If taking a clinical exam, are the examiners looking for demonstrating a structured examination technique or is making the correct diagnosis an essential requirement?
- Identify relevant exam related courses and apply for these well in advance, as popular ones are often oversubscribed. Look around as course quality may vary. The amount of learning such courses can provide may be invaluable.

- You may be highly competent and safe, in doing your day to day job, but that may not be enough for passing exams. Exams aim to test knowledge and skills required not only for commonly encountered scenarios but also for the unusual rare ones. Examine the syllabus to be tested and work though that in a systematic way.
- Speak to those who previously sat the exam. What questions did they get? How did they revise? Which courses did they find relevant and useful? Speak to those who flew through the exam, and those who failed it or encountered difficulties. What do they think went wrong?
- Inform your senior colleagues at work about your upcoming exam and ask them to quiz you and test you in clinics, ward rounds, and theatres.
- Ask your peers and seniors to let you know if they see any unusual or interesting clinical signs in clinic or ward.
- Service provision, learning, and exam preparation, are not mutually exclusive. Try and treat those clinical cases you encounter daily in your practise as an exam case. If you take a history and clinically assess a patient in clinic, try and do so as if you were in an exam. It is unlikely it will take much longer, and, if anything, it may make your clerking more structured. In presenting that case to your senior, do so as if talking to an examiner. In describing a radiograph use the approach you would use in an exam.
- Get in study groups. Find peers who are also preparing for the exam, and arrange to meet at regular intervals, share knowledge, discuss poorly understood topics, or examine patients in front of each other. Be prepared to give and receive feedback.
- Know your strengths and also weaknesses. When revising, concentrate on the things you are not good at, rather than on those you are confident. Concentrate on your weaknesses rather than your strengths. Breath of knowledge is as important as detailed knowledge in exams.
- Study exam related books.
- Access candidates' discussion forums on the internet. What questions were asked before?
- Consider taking a few days off work before the exam, to rest and focus your thoughts. Sitting an exam after a night on call, may not be the best option.
- If a clinical exam is organised at your hospital offer to help, even if it is still a long time ahead for you to do that exam. It may give you insight on how examiners think, what types of cases are chosen, how different candidates perform.
- Enjoy the revision. In the medical school you may have to study and pass exams in areas of Medicine which might not greatly interest you. Postgraduate exams are usually in an area you have chosen as a prospective career, and hence revising and getting better at it, should be enjoyable.

Postgraduate Degrees

As part of your postgraduate learning and training you may consider doing a post-graduate degree. A wide variety of options are available varying from Diplomas, to Masters, to Doctorates. Such degrees may be, amongst others, in a clinical, scientific, research, or teaching area. Postgraduate degrees maybe part time, or full time.

Reasons for doing a post-graduate degree:

1. Gain more knowledge in a clinical or scientific area that interests you.
2. There is a subject you are very passionate about and want to study in detail.
3. Gain research experience.
4. Develop skills not easily acquired in your working environment (teaching, managerial).
5. Improve your CV and aid career progression.
6. May be an essential requirement of your training program for career progression.

Consider carefully as to whether to undertake such a task, when you want to do it, and in what area. Postgraduate Degrees can offer an invaluable experience. Like professional exams, postgraduate degrees, may provide you with a qualification to stay with you for ever. Job titles and appointments may not exist or have the same weight in different parts of the world, as degrees do.

Teaching

Those who know, do. Those that understand, teach

Aristotle [1]

As a doctor you may be involved in teaching. You may be involved in bed site teaching, formal teaching, one to one, small group teaching, large group teaching. If taking on a teaching role consider the following:

- Understand the aims of your learners, what they are aiming to gain, and gear the teaching to that. One way, is asking the students at the beginning what they are trying to get out of the session, as a guide of what you should aim to present.

    - If you are teaching at an exam revision course the attendants are likely to be looking at potential exam questions and answers, rather than a long detailed explanation of facts that are not part of the exam syllabus.
    - If you are teaching fractures to Emergency Department juniors it is likely they will be looking for methods of splinting and plastering for when fractures first present, rather than the details of complex surgical fixation.

- Establish what the starting knowledge of the learners is and build on that. If the learner is not aware of the basics and principles, there is little scope jumping to the complex stuff.
- Engage the audience through questions, or assigned tasks. Try and include all, not just the very proactive ones. If you are to question go round the group, rather than concentrating on the person offering the answer every time.
- Try and teach principles rather than mere facts. Help the learner to work out the answer. Bring examples from their previous experiences and use them to help solve new problems.
- Respect those you are teaching, do not make them feel uncomfortable for lack of knowledge. Get to know their names, level of training, get an interest in them.
- Consider testing, both prior to and after delivery of teaching, to see what the learners have gained.
- Give teaching that you enjoy, topics that you know well.
- If you do not know the answer to a question, promise to look it up and get back to them. Alternatively, agree with the student for both of you to seek the answer and discuss it at a later stage. It is not difficult to see when someone is guessing the answer and that could affect your credibility, even for facts you truly know. A teacher does not have to know all.
- Attend formal teaching courses, to improve your teaching skills.
- Devote time to preparation.
- Teach by example, as juniors and trainees learn lots through observation of behaviours and actions. Put your best performance in front of them, in how you deal with patients, colleagues, situations and problems. Juniors may look at you as a role model and their impressions may be long lasting.

- Test that your message is getting across. Give facts, and then question the learner as to what they understand. Show a procedure and then ask them to demonstrate it back. A learner nodding at what you say may not be one who fully understands.
- Demonstrate the limitations of what you are teaching. Make it clear when knowledge is grey, rather than trying to paint it all black or white.
- Be considerate to the patient, respect their confidentiality, ask for permission to involve them in teaching, consider asking for their feedback.
- Continuously evaluate your teaching methods. Either by feedback from the trainees, or colleagues and other peers. This will help you further develop your training methods, but may also help you gather evidence for you professional development.
- Do not view questions or queries by the students as doubting your knowledge or authority. If you explained something but it is not understood, knowing that may help you rethink how to present it next time. Questions may also help you reconsider concepts you long thought were clear and obvious. We often learn from our trainees as much as they learn from us.
- Give handouts to facilitate attention, so that learners do not spend all time making notes. Allow space in handouts to take limited additional notes. Handouts with your slides would of value. Be aware of copyright regulations in distributing copied work.
- Provide specific advise about further reading (textbooks, articles).

Many of us may still recall an outstanding teacher from our early school days, someone we respect, admire and on occasions miss. We may recall a trainer at university or postgraduate training that we saw as a role model, someone we hoped to match one day. How did that teacher or trainer behave, why was that teacher inspiring? As a teacher now yourself, what behaviours can you adopt to infuse those feelings to your students or trainees?

Lecturing

Lectures form a vital part of medical education as they allow a large volume of factual information to be conveyed to large groups of learners. Lectures can be of great value or of minimal educational value, depending on how they are delivered and how the message gets across.

In giving a lecture consider:

- Give a clear aim as to what the lecture aims to achieve.
- Give a plan of your lecture, outlining the structure of your presentation. Set the layout of lecture with planned breaks.
- Keep it simple, use easily understood language.
- You may not be able to provide all essential information or give detailed facts as part of the lecture, but can give pointers as to where to find that information. These may be articles or books for further reference.
- Use repetition for important concepts. Use different ways of explaining one concept to ensure the message gets across.
- There are several techniques to maintain interest and attention throughout lectures. It has been shown that the maximum attention during a lecture (as assessed by note taking) is within the first 15 min, with concentration levels gradually declining after that, only to go up again towards the end [16, 17] (Fig. 5.4). Hence, avoid very long lectures, and give your important messages early on, or leave them till the very end. Try to arouse interest at regular intervals, to re-start the attention curve. Several techniques may be used to engage the audience, encourage active learning, and stimulate attention [18, 19]. These may include:

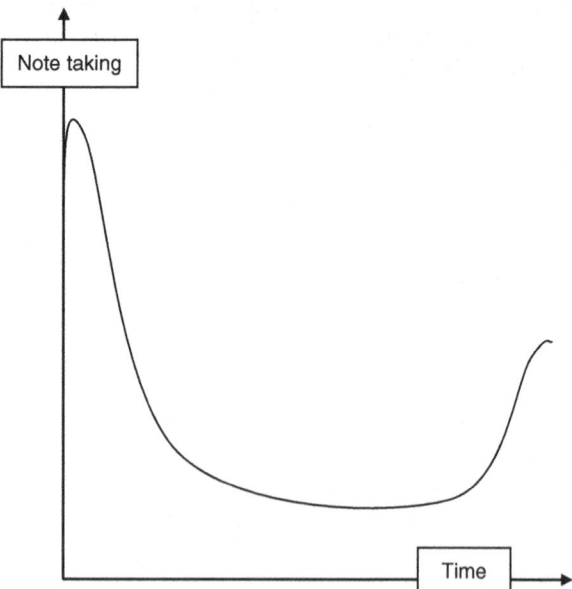

Fig. 5.4 Fluctuation of note taking, as a marker of learners' attention, during a lecture over time (Adapted from Bligh [17])

1. Questioning
2. Brainstorming
3. Small group discussions
4. Problem solving
5. Peer teaching
6. Role playing
7. Regular breaks, stand up, stretch legs

• Summarise at the end of the lecture, stressing important take home messages. If students were to remember one single thing from the lecture, which one would that be?

Assessing Trainees

Everybody is a genius. But if you judge a fish by its ability to climb a tree, it will live its whole life believing that it is stupid

Albert Einstein [1]

There may be a structured assessment process that you need to familiarise yourself with. Devote time to giving feedback, respect the assessment process. The trainee may have put all the effort and preparation for this assessment, and your part is to give it the attention it deserves.

- Give positive feedback followed by constructive criticisms.
- Give feedback soon after the assessment process.
- Describe the good and not so good things you observed.
- Described what you observed in detail, rather than simply giving an overall impression, to allow the individual to specifically learn.
- Give details for areas of improvement.
- Have a clear understanding in the assessment tools and get trained in them. If a formal assessment process or evaluation tools are not available, consider using Miller's pyramid [20] (Fig. 5.5). This provides a structure for assessing clinical competence. It describes the various clinical competencies in four stages as "knows", "knows how", "demonstrates" and "does". "Does" refers to action taken in real practise.
- View assessment tools as a way of putting structure to the assessment process, rather than another piece of paperwork.

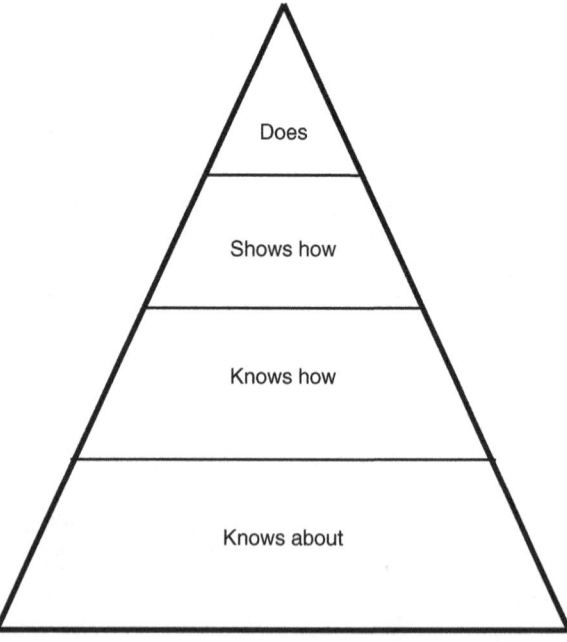

Fig. 5.5 Miller's pyramid of assessment (Adapted from Miller [20])

Organising a Course

As a doctor you may organise a medical course or a workshop, as part of your training activities. Organising a successful course is a challenging task that requires careful thought, planning and preparation. In organising a course consider the following;

- Need –
  - Is there a true need for the course?
  - What is this course trying to achieve? Address a local audience, fill a vacuum of courses on the topic to be covered, improve on content and style of an existing course?

- Audience –
  - Who will be the target audience? Will it be local, regional, national or international?
  - Level of training? Is it aimed at medical students, junior doctors, senior doctors or allied health professionals?
  - How many attendants aimed at? What if too many or too few apply?

- Why would the audience attend? Will they attend aiming to aid exam preparation, improve knowledge or develop new skills?
- Format – What will the format be? Will it be lectures, small group discussions or practical workshops?
- Location – Where will it take place, what facilities are necessary and what are available?
- Faculty –
  - Who will deliver the course?
  - Availability of faculty?
  - Interest and reliability in participating?

- Costs –
  - Paying for venue, administrative support, faculty attendance or travel, adverts.
  - Sponsors?
  - Delegates paying fee? If course is free, how can attendance be ensured? Paying fee to be returned upon attendance may facilitate attendance.

- Timing of course – Is it clashing with other courses? Is it in time for upcoming exams, holidays, faculty availability?
- Accommodation – For faculty or attendees. Will this be provided as part of the course fee? Can a list of local accommodation facilities be constructed?
- Advertisement – How will the course be advertised?
- Plan in advance.

- Advertise in advance but also closer to the course.
- Confirm faculty attendance well in advance.

- Registration process – Have a clearly identified contact person for attendees and faculty.
- Involvement of patients – How will they be identified and asked for participation, travel to and from hospital?
- Course material – Printouts, booklets.
- Feedback – Obtain feedback at end of the course and use it to improve further courses.

References

1. Famous quotes at brainyquote. www.brainyquote.com. Accessed on 23 Sept 2014.
2. Dunn R, Dunn K. Using learning styles data to develop student prescriptions. In: Keefe JW, editor. Student learning styles diagnosing and prescribing programs. Reston: National Association of Secondary School Principals; 1979.
3. Dunn R, Dunn K. Teaching elementary students through their individual learning styles. Boston: Allyn & Bacon; 1992.
4. Kolb D. Experiential learning: experience as the source of learning and development. Englewood Cliffs: Prentice Hall; 1984.
5. Banning M. Approaches to teaching: current opinions and related research. Nurse Educ Today. 2005;25(7):502–8.
6. Masters K. Edgar Dale's pyramid of learning in medical education: a literature review. Med Teach. 2013;35(11):e1584–93.
7. Lalley JP, Miller RH. The learning pyramid: does it point teachers in the right direction? Education. 2007;128(1):64–79.
8. Hjortdah P, Laerum E. Continuity of care in general practice: effect on patient satisfaction. BMJ. 1992;304(6837):1287–90.
9. The free dictionary. http://www.thefreedictionary.com. Accessed on 25 Sept 2014.
10. Akhtar KS, Chen A, Standfield NJ, Gupte CM. The role of simulation in developing surgical skills. Curr Rev Musculoskelet Med. 2014;7(2):155–60.
11. Herrmann-Werner A, Nikendei C, Keifenheim K, Bosse HM, Lund F, Wagner R, Celebi N, Zipfel S, Weyrich P. "Best practice" skills lab training vs. a "see one, do one" approach in undergraduate medical education: an RCT on students' long-term ability to perform procedural clinical skills. PLoS ONE. 2013;8(9):e76354. doi:10.1371/journal.pone.0076354.
12. Birnbaumer DM. Teaching procedures: improving "see one, do one, teach one". CJEM. 2011;13(6):390–4.
13. Lenchus JD. End of the "see one, do one, teach one" era: the next generation of invasive bedside procedural instruction. J Am Osteopath Assoc. 2010;110(6):340–6.
14. Rodriguez-Paz JM, Kennedy M, Salas E, Wu AW, Sexton JB, Hunt EA, Pronovost PJ. Beyond "see one, do one, teach one": toward a different training paradigm. Postgrad Med J. 2009;85(1003):244–9.
15. Mason WT, Strike PW. See one, do one, teach one–is this still how it works? A comparison of the medical and nursing professions in the teaching of practical procedures. Med Teach. 2003;25(6):664–6.
16. Lloyd D. A concept of improvement of learning response in the taught lesson. Vis Educ. 1968;34:23–5.
17. Bligh D. What's the use of lectures? 5th ed. England, UK: Intellect, Exeter; 1998.
18. Ruhl KL, Suritsky S. The pause procedure and/or an outline. Effect on immediate free recall and lecture notes taken by college students with learning disabilities. Learn Disabil Q. 1995;18(1):2–11. Winter.
19. Weaver RL, Cotrell HW. Mental aerobics: the half sheet response. Innov High Educ. 1985;10(1):23–31.
20. Miller GE. The assessment of clinical skills/competence/performance. Acad Med. 1990;65(9 Suppl):S63–7.

Chapter 6
Procedural Skills

As a doctor you may have to perform practical medical procedures which may vary from technically simple to technically complex tasks. No matter how technically simple a procedure may seem, it is still a significant event for a patient and should hence be approached as such.

Procedures may be carried out in clinic, ward or theatre, in community or hospital settings. Some procedures are widely used by doctors of various specialties (cannulation, catheterisation, venepuncture, joint injection or aspiration), whilst some are more specialty or sub-specialty specific (intubation, chest drain insertion, fracture reduction and fixation).

Being able to learn and perform a procedure is a skill to be developed, whatever the procedure may be. Like other tasks, procedural skills have a learning curve. The slope of such learning curve may be influenced by the procedure per se, but also by the planning, effort, training and perseverance of the operator.

This chapter describes a cycle of procedural learning, and discusses what one must consider prior to, during, and after carrying out a procedure. An outline as how to document invasive procedures is also given.

© Springer International Publishing Switzerland 2015
C. Panayiotou Charalambous, *Career Skills for Doctors*,
DOI 10.1007/978-3-319-13479-6_6

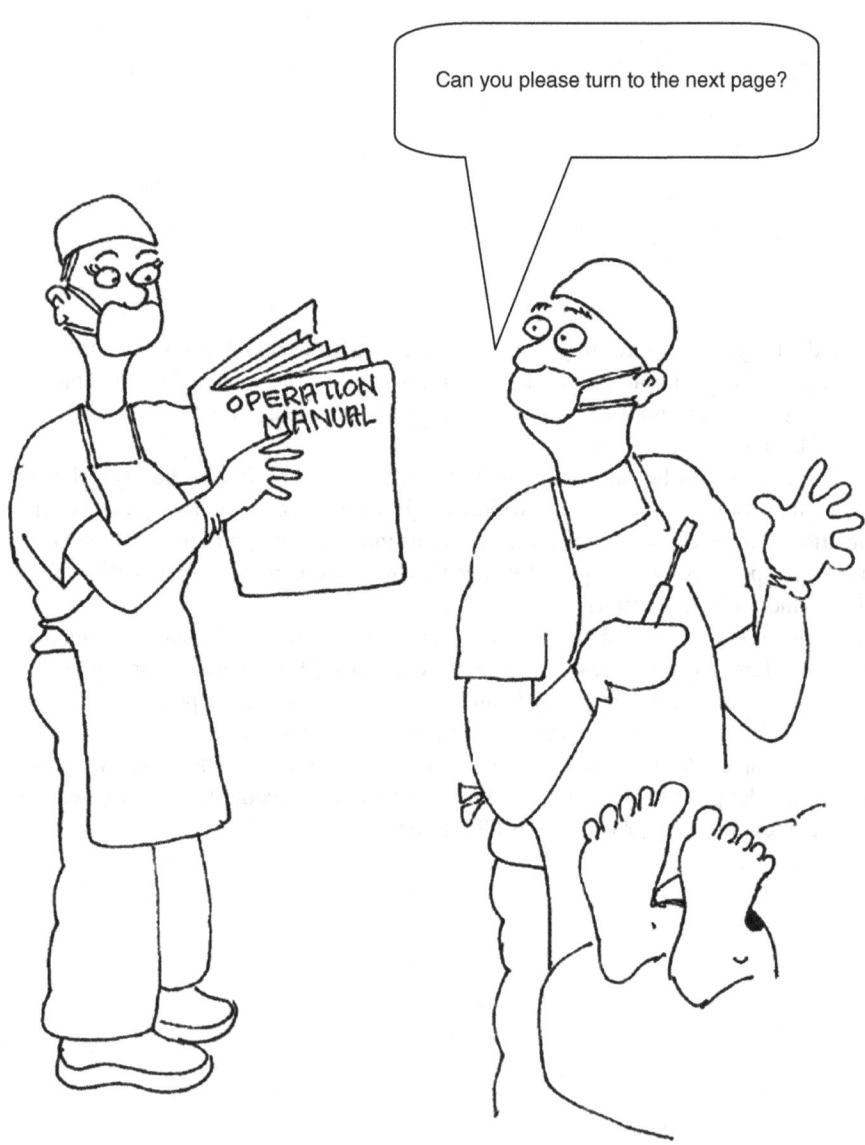

Learning a Procedure

A long apprenticeship is the most logical way to success

Chet Atkins [1]

Becoming able to carry out a medical procedure is, to some extent, equivalent to mastering any other technical skill. It requires knowledge, but also manual dexterity. In developing a procedural skill the cycle of procedural learning LOAD (Fig. 6.1) may be applied. LOAD describes the essential steps in acquiring a new technical skill and stands for:

L-earn about the procedure – initially using passive ways of learning- reading, lectures.
O-bserve the procedure – watch the video, watch in real life.
A-ssist in the procedure – as a first or otherwise assistant, in simulator or real life.
D-o the procedure – in simulator or real life, in full or in small progressive steps.

In going through the LOAD cycle for a particular procedure, consider the following:

- Make the best of every training opportunity. Observe different practitioners performing the same procedure. Learn from the skilled and less so skilled. What could you have done differently? What would an alternative approach be?
- When it comes to hands on experience simulation may be of high value, both in assisting or carrying out the procedure. Simulation allows you to practise and make mistakes, without worrying about any actual harm to the patient.
- For complex lengthy procedures break the procedure into smaller components, and learn how to do those one at a time. Once you master each step, you may then proceed to performing the whole of the procedure.
- Even though LOAD refers to a progressive cycle of procedural learning, one may need to go back and forth. In particular, once you start doing the procedure go back and read about it. Similarly go back and again observe or assist someone

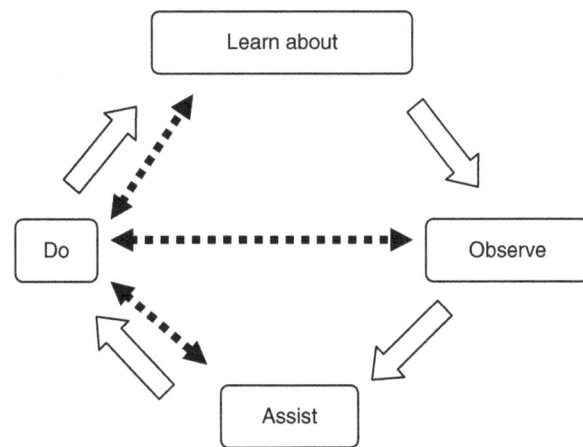

Fig. 6.1 Procedural learning cycle – LOAD

else doing it, to help you clarify queries arisen whilst doing the procedure your-self. Hence, assisting in a procedure you are able to do, is itself of educational value.

- When you start doing the procedure do so with a more senior assisting you or closely supervising you. Build your confidence in doing the procedure, gradually doing it under less and less supervision, before undertaking the task completely on your own.
- Develop alternative approaches, as a backup, if a procedure does not go accord-ing to your initial plan. Anticipate and prepare as how to deal with complica-tions. Discuss with more experienced operators what complications they have encountered, and how they dealt with them.

Preparing for a Procedure

I would like to see the day when somebody would be appointed surgeon somewhere who had no hands, for the operative part is the least part of the work

Harvey Cushing [2]

Being able to carry out a medical procedure is not simply about inserting the cannula, inserting the urinary catheter, stitching the bowel, screwing the bone. In doing a procedure one must take into account the patient as a whole, as well as the environment in which the procedure takes place. In learning, observing, assisting or doing a procedure you may consider:

- Indications for performing the procedure.

  - Is the procedure needed?
  - Is an alternative available?

- Resources needed – equipment, staff.

  - Equipment – what equipment do you need? Type and size of suture, type and size of urinary catheter, what cannula will you use?
  - Know your instruments and equipment. You are in charge of a procedure you are doing. Do not rely on the ward nurse, the scrub nurse, or theatre staff, for passing you the correct instruments or knowing which instruments to use. It maybe they are new too, they may not have been involved in this procedure before. You are in lead, you are in charge, you need to know your instruments to guide the rest.
  - Availability of your instruments – Are they still on the shelf or have they run out? Should you get them nearby to avoid running back and forth?
  - Sterilisation of your instruments before you start- Are the equipment sterilised, has the sterilisation run out of date, is there a breach to the sterilisation pack?
  - What staff do you need? What assistants? How skilled does the assistant has to be?
  - Equipment support – do you need the equipment company representative to be there, if using new unfamiliar equipment?

- Anaesthetic issues –

  - Local, general, regional?
  - Is anaesthetist available?
  - Is anaesthetist able to deliver what you expect? Able to intubate an infant, do a specialised nerve block?

- Patient preparation

  - Bowel preparation
  - Anxiolytic

- Patient consenting

  - Written
  - Verbal

- Positioning

  - How will you position the patient?
  - Where will you stand, where will the assistant stand?
  - If under X-Ray control which way will the image intensifier approach the operating table?
  - What operating table will you need? Is it radiolucent?

- Draping

  - Cloth, disposable
  - Extent of draping

- Haemostasis – how will you minimise bleeding?

  - Tourniquette
  - Diathermy
  - Local adrenaline
  - Controlled hypotension

- Infection prevention

  - Prepping
  - Antibiotic prophylaxis
  - Operator's clothing

- Thrombo-prophylaxis

  - Mechanical
  - Chemical

- Physiological parameters

  - Glycemic control
  - Temperature

- Wound dressings

  - Bandage?
  - Splint or sling?

- Post procedure management

  - Monitoring
  - Anaesthetic wearing off
  - Mobilisation, commencement of eating
  - Wound inspection, discharge

Doing the Procedure

When it comes to the procedure it self, a structured approach is needed. You may split the procedure into:

Approach

- Which part of the body?
- What skin incision is required?
- What are the planes of deeper dissection?

Procedure steps

- Core of procedure

Wound closure

- What layers to close?
- How to close them?

The following may help you go through the procedure:

- Plan who will do what. What will you be doing? What will your assistant be doing?

  - If cannulating, an assistant may calm and distract the patient.
  - If catheterising, an assistant may open and pass you the catheter and other equipment.
  - If reducing a fracture, an assistant may counteract your pull.
  - If removing an appendix, an assistant may retract the soft tissues.

- Know your anatomy – Normal and variations.
- Keep it simple – Avoid converting a simple task into a complex multi-step procedure. The outcome matters more than the complexity of getting there.
- Learn what you can accept.

  - The vein you cannulated is small and thin – can you accept that or do you need to look for another one?
  - The screw you inserted is not central in the bone –can you accept that or does it need repositioning?
  - The chest drain is not reaching the lung apex. Can you accept that or does it need further insertion?

- Which are the essential steps, which can you skip?
- The learning curve relies not only on the technique or steps of the procedure but also on the use of specific instruments. When new instruments are used, a new learning curve may apply. Use instruments you are familiar with. Avoid keep altering the equipment you use, unless there is a good reason.

Post Procedure

After participating in a procedure, reflect on what was done and what has been learnt. What was done well, what could have been done better? Make notes, write down what you observed or what you did. Every time you are involved in a similar procedure you can add further notes as to what else you have learnt. This can help put a structure to your learning, but also act as a revision tool prior to doing the procedure again. Document the procedure in a structured way. Follow the patient through. How did the patient do? Any complications related to the procedure?

Recording Invasive Procedures

Whether inserting a urinary catheter in a ward patient, administering a steroid injection in clinic, inserting an arterial line in critical care, or carrying out complex surgery in theatre, a record of performing an invasive procedure should be clearly made. By recording this you are communicating what the procedure was, why the procedure was carried out, what happened during the procedure, and what the post-procedure plan is. This communication is particularly important in continuity of care, such as if a complication of the procedure arose, but such documentation is often poor [3, 4]. The exact length, format, and subheadings of a procedure record may vary according to your working environment, and the procedure per se, but this could include:

- Title of procedure.
- Anatomical site (including left/right if applicable).
- Date and time of procedure.
- Indication (such as acute retention, fracture).
- Details of operator.
- Details of assistant, scrub nurse, anaesthetist.
- Method of anaesthesia.
- Aseptic precautions.
- Position of patient.
- Tourniquet use, antibiotic prophylaxis, thrombo-prophylaxis, bowel preparation.
- Skin incision, deeper exposure.
- Findings.
- Procedure – stepwise description of what was performed.
- Closure of wound – types of sutures used per layer, method of suturing, glue or clip usage.
- Post procedure instructions (antibiotics, timing of reduction of dressing and wound inspection, conditions to be satisfied for removing chest drain or wound drain, thrombo-prophylaxis, timing of suture removal, mobilisation status, physiotherapy, postoperative diet, further procedures needed is symptoms do not improve, discharge plans, follow up appointment).
- Details and signature of person documenting procedure.

References

1. Famous Quotes at BrainyQuote. www.brainyquote.com. Accessed on 23 Sept 14.
2. Wikiquote. http://en.wikiquote.org/wiki/Surgery. Accessed on 25 Sept 14.
3. Tijani KH, Lawal AO, Ojewola RW, Badmus TA. Quality of documentation of urethral catheterization in a Nigerian teaching hospital. Niger Q J Hosp Med. 2010;20(4):177–80.
4. Conybeare A, Pathak S, Imam I. The quality of hospital records of urethral catheterisation. Ann R Coll Surg Engl. 2002;84(2):109–10.

Chapter 7
Research and Audit

Research is defined by the Oxford dictionary as "the systematic investigation into and study of materials and sources in order to establish facts and reach new conclusions" [1]. Clinical audit is defined as "a quality improvement process that seeks to improve patient care and outcomes through systematic review of care against explicit criteria and the implementation of change" [2].

In clinical practise research may be considered as the process through which we try to determine what the ideal practise is. In contrast, in audit the ideal practise is known and we try to determine whether our current practise meets that ideal.

Participation in research and audit may form integral components of a doctor's training and practise. They are important in advancing knowledge and improving the quality of care we provide.

This chapter aims to answer commonly asked questions about research and audit and help you develop the necessary related research and audit skills.

© Springer International Publishing Switzerland 2015
C. Panayiotou Charalambous, *Career Skills for Doctors*,
DOI 10.1007/978-3-319-13479-6_7

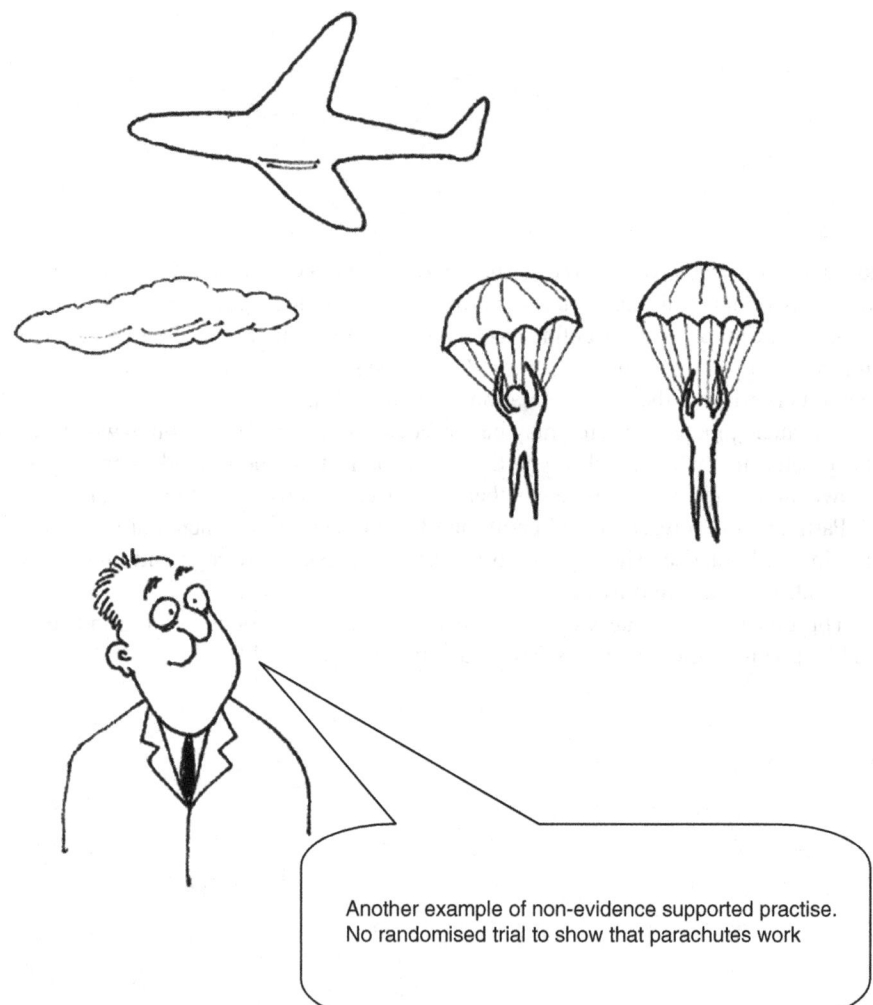

Should Clinicians Get Involved in Research?

Research is creating new knowledge

Neil Armstrong [3]

Research is the process through which new developments and discoveries are made, and through which knowledge advances. Clinicians are often in a central position of understanding the clinical needs for new developments. Hence, clinicians are vital in driving clinical improvement innovations and this can be achieved through participation in research.

As clinicians we are practising in the era of evidence based Medicine, whereby we aim to use the best available evidence in guiding us to provide high quality clinical care. We must thus be able to analyse and interpret the available published evidence, and draw clear conclusions based on that. Carrying out research may allow you to gain first hand experience with regards the challenges and limitations of research, and hence place you in a better position for critically appraising the available evidence. It helps you appreciate that our knowledge and understanding is often not black or white, but somewhere in a gray zone in between.

The problem solving skills and thought provoking processes required for research, may provide you with enjoyment and stimulation other than that gained from direct clinical care.

Patients are increasingly becoming aware of research, and patient driven research is on the rise. Even if you are not carrying out research projects yourself, your patients may want to discuss ongoing national or international studies and the merits of entering those.

Participation in research may be essential for career progression. Carrying out research and publishing your work may give extra weight to your CV, making you more competitive for job applications.

Research paper interpretation and analysis is often an integral part of postgraduate exams and assessments, and participation in research helps further develop such skills.

When to Do Research?

The best time to plant a tree was 20 years ago. The second best time is now
Chinese proverb [4]

You can get involved in research at any stage of your career. It is never too early
or too late. As long as you can put the effort, and devote the time, you may take
it on.

- As an undergraduate you may get involved in research, through research mod-
  ules or electives at medical school. You may join ongoing research projects of
  your science or clinical supervisors alongside your university studies.
- You may take a year out from medical school studies intercalating in a basic science or other degree, which has a research component.
- You may think of research at postgraduate level when considering your next job
  application, and you are trying to further improve your CV.
- You may look into research when you become aware that it is a requirement of
  your postgraduate training program.
- You may decide early on in your career that you want to become a clinical academic, where research forms a large part of your work practise.
- You may consider research at a later stage in your career, as a break from or as a
  complement of clinical work.
- You may consider research post retirement from clinical work, to use the knowledge and experience accumulated over the years to identify questions that may
  be answered through research.

Decide why you want to get involved and whether you can give it what is needed.
Any time can be a good time for research.

What Type of Research? How Big Project?

If you can't do great things, do small things in a great way

Napoleon Hill [3]

Research may be basic science, clinical research (bed site, translational, epidemiological), or literature based. It may be part time research, alongside your main clinical work, or full time, with no clinical work attached. You may do a research post with some clinical sessions to maintain a clinical touch.

In deciding what type of research to do, or how big project to take, you may consider:

- How much time are you prepared to devote? How much time will you realistically be able to devote? Can you devote a fixed regular time, or are you looking for more flexibility?
- What are you aiming to achieve? Understand research principles, publish, boost your CV, or making a huge discovery?
- What research options are available? This may be available by your supervisors, your institution, your local universities.
- Can it be seen through? Taking on a simple project that stands a good chance of completion and publication, in your allocated time, may be better than a much larger complex project, which you are unlikely to complete. When applying for a new job or post, many interview marking schemes have marks allocation for research, according to its stage of progress. A completed project may score higher that one in the pipeline. Published (or accepted for publication) research, may score more than research that has yet to be analysed and submitted for publication.
- Is it relevant to your needs? If planning to become a brain surgeon, should you be looking into a research project in neurosurgery rather than gynaecology?
- Is your research needed? What will your research findings add? Will your research provide something novel or original? A similar study may have already been done, but repeating it may be of value in validating previously reported results, or in assessing how one intervention behaves in different settings.

If a project does not seem right for you, if you feel you may not be able to complete it, be honest and say so at the beginning. Giving promises you know you may not be able to keep, is not fair on those who may be able to offer that research project to someone else. Similarly, if you are considering what projects to allocate to your juniors, consider meeting with them, see what they are aiming to achieve, how much time they can devote, how much experience of research they have (a copy of their CV could help) and then allocate a realistic project.

Will the Chosen Research Be Good Enough?

Do what you can, where you are, with what you have

Teddy Roosevelt [3]

Will you research be good enough, valued as high quality research?

For clinical studies, the quality of research may be summarised according to the quality of evidence it provides. Multiple schemes for describing levels of evidence exist [5–7] but these could be simply described as the Research Ladder (Fig. 7.1). In the Research Ladder description of personal opinions is the first step, climbing on to reporting single or limited number of clinical cases, retrospective studies (such as case-control studies), prospective studies (such as cohort studies), randomised controlled trials and finally systematic reviews and meta-analyses. This order of ascending is however not absolute. A well designed large prospective cohort study may give better evidence than a small, poorly designed randomised controlled trial. A randomised controlled trial may give more reliable information than a meta-analysis of several cohort studies.

When you enter research, you may start at the bottom of the Research Ladder or jump to any other step. It is a skill to realise that any research may give valuable information, no matter how small it seems. We initially develop thoughts and concepts or make noticeable observations, before we embark on testing them with large trials. Hence, expression of opinions or description of isolated observations has a merit of its own. Randomised controlled trials are often considered the gold standard of clinical research [8]. However, resources, practicalities and ethics may not allow us to address every question with a randomised trial, and other designs may be more practical and acceptable. Do not rush to dismiss a project, as it is not high up in the ladder. When you initially try to develop your research skills, the review of a case report or small case series maybe a reasonable starting step. It may help you develop skills of study design, data collection, analysis, making sound conclusions, manuscript preparation, presentation and submission for publication.

Is it better to have completed a research project, no matter how small it may seem, or wait for the huge idea or the best trial to come along? Is it better to put a step on the ladder, or simply sit on the side watching others ascend?

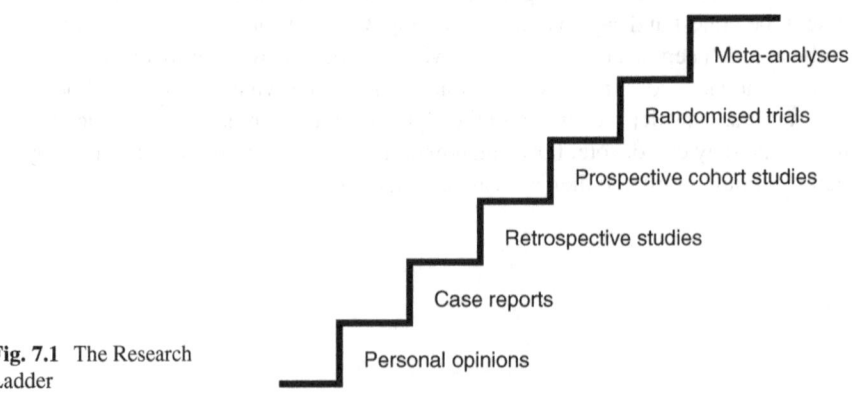

Fig. 7.1 The Research Ladder

Who to Do Research With?

Personal brands are determined by a track record of actions, not a track record of plans
Ryan Lilly [3]

When considering as to who to do research with, there are certain factors to consider, depending on what you aim to achieve. It maybe that you are at the beginning of your career, aiming to get a basic understanding of research principles. It maybe that you want to join a research program, to complete a postgraduate degree through a research thesis. It maybe that you want to research a specific topic, close to your heart, and in which you want to make a real contribution. It maybe that you want to do research in a world known institution, to strengthen your CV and aid career progression. It maybe that you want to get published for improving your chances at the next job application. Location may be a factor. You may be looking for research close to home, or a project that can be done from home.

Before committing your self to a particular research program, supervisor, or collaborator, explore what is available. Seek information and advice from colleagues, who may have done research previously, or may have worked with the group you want to join. Meet the potential research lead, to discuss what you are aiming to gain from your research, and whether that could be met through their research program. Some of the factors you may need to consider:

- Will you get the necessary support and supervision? Will your project get the time and attention you are looking for?
- Is it feasible to be done given the time constraints?
- Is funding needed and if so is it available?
- Will you enjoy working with your potential collaborators?
- Will the proposed project lead to a successful thesis?
- Is your research likely to get published? If your aim is to get published it would be reasonable to check your potential supervisor with regards to their publication track record, and the web makes that easy. How many articles have they published, what journals did they publish in, when was the last time they published? If you want to learn how to auscultate heart murmurs you would join a cardiologist's clinic; if you want to get published should you not be joining someone with a high publication output?

Research Process

The process of research may be described in the form of the Research Cycle (Fig. 7.2). It involves developing a research idea, reviewing the available literature to determine what is already known, identifying areas that need further investigation, and formulating a clear aim as to what the new research aims to achieve. This is followed by designing and delivering the methodology that will allow the research question to be answered. This involves data collection, analysis and interpretation. Conclusions based on findings are then made, and new areas that need further investigation are identified, leading to further research, and hence a new beginning of the Research Cycle.

Research idea The research idea may be yours, or someone else's, your supervisor's, your juniors', your patients'. In reviewing the literature you need to determine what is known about the subject, has your question been investigated before, what new could you be adding? Search medical search engines/databases (such as the National Library of Medicine, National Health System Evidence, Excerpta Medica) and also general search engines (such as Google, Yahoo, AltaVista). Initially carry out a broad search, to avoid missing out relevant information. Based on what you find, you may decide whether to further pursue your research idea or not. Even if your idea has already been tested you may still pursue it, to validate or dispute previously reported results, use methodology that will give more robust results (better design, larger sample size), or determine whether findings can be applied in different contexts and populations.

Aims Based on what you are planning to investigate formulate your research question, and clearly state your aims. If you have more than one aim, clarify which is the primary and which are the secondary objectives.

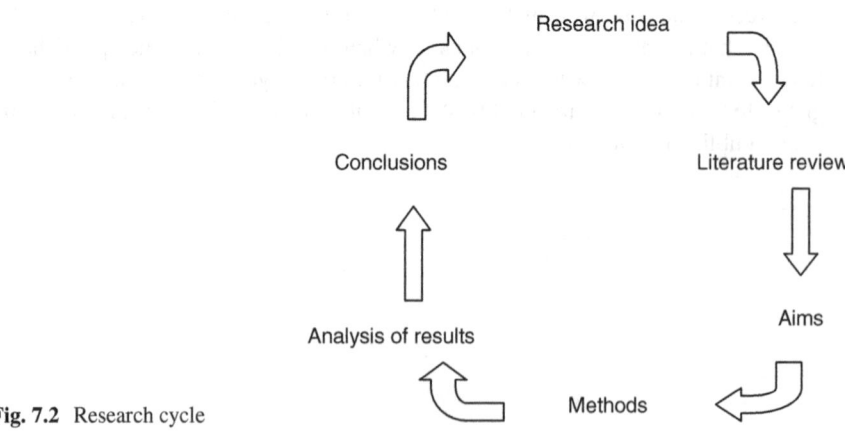

Fig. 7.2 Research cycle

Methods Choose the appropriate methodology that will allow you to answer your question, taking into account the resources you have available. This includes study design, ethical issues, costs (time, personnel, other resources).

Study design With regards to study design, this will depend on the specifics of your research project. For clinical research you may consider:

- Prospective/retrospective study?
- Catchment population, identification and recruitment of participants, inclusion and exclusion criteria.
- Sample size. How many participants will you need to demonstrate the presence or confirm the absence of differences amongst groups? Which of the outcomes is used to estimate sample size? Can such samples be achieved?
- How will the intervention be applied?
- What outcomes will be assessed and how?
- Will the participants, researchers and analysts be blinded with regards interventions administered?
- How will bias be minimised or avoided?

Research team Define the members of the research team and their specific roles and responsibilities. The exact team members will vary, depending on the research study, and may include:

- Medical personnel.
- Research nurses.
- Allied health care professionals.
- Basic scientists.
- Statistician.
- Health economist.
- Lay person.
- Administrators.
- Research manager.

Analysis and presentation of results Collected data will need to be analysed to aid understanding and interpretation. They will then have to be presented in a suitable, easily understood form (written, tabular, graphic). You may consider:

- Decide in advance how results will be analysed and presented, but re-examine whether given the data collected the exact analysis needs to be reconsidered.
- Are data quantitative or qualitative?
- Will the raw data or variables calculated from the raw data, be used in analysis?
- How will participants lost to follow or dropping out of the study be dealt with in the analysis?
- Are you looking for a difference between groups in any direction, or do you know which direction the results will go?

Interpretations and conclusions   Once analysed, data are examined, interpreted and conclusions made. Consider:

- What do the analysed results show?
- What is the significance of the findings?
- Are the results expected or surprising?
- Does statistical significance equate to clinical importance?
- How far can the findings be extrapolated?
- What are the limitations of the results obtained?
- Are the aims of the study met?
- What new questions arise?
- What further research is needed?

Research Ethics   As part of the methodology you need to consider research ethics. The Declaration of Helsinki (developed by the World Medical Association) was described initially in 1964 and has since been revised on multiple occasions. It is a set of ethical principles regarding human research [9] and is considered the gold standard on human research ethics. Various professional associations, government bodies, healthcare research institutions, universities, and funding bodies, have also developed codes of research practise and ethics [10–13]. In designing your study you must ensure that the rights of research participants are protected and their well being, safety, and dignity are respected. Some ethical issues to consider are:

- Do any potential benefits of the proposed research outweigh any risks to participants?
- What measures are taken to minimise risk of harm to participants and what actions will be taken if that were to happen? What compensation arrangements are in place?
- Will vulnerable patients (children, people with learning disabilities or diminished cognition) be included, and what specific measures are taken to protect them?
- How will informed consent be secured? How will participants be given clear information to allow informed consent for entering the study? What about patients who can not give informed consent?
- How will participants' confidentiality be protected, and how will data collected be secured? What will be the period of data retention?
- How will funding sources, researchers' affiliations, or conflicting interests, be declared? What measures are taken to ensure that these do not influence the conduct of research, or the report of its outcomes?
- What measures are taken to ensure outcomes are disseminated no matter what they are?
- What measures are taken to ensure researches are properly trained and competent in conducting research?

Approvals   What approvals are necessary for your research to start? You may need your institutions research review board approval, Ethics committee review and approval, service and financial managers' approval. Make a list of what is needed and get them early.

Obtaining Funding for Research

Research studies can be costly with regards staffing costs, capital expenses, disposables. How will the research be funded? There are several sources for obtaining research funding and include:

- Research charities.
- Training overseeing bodies such as medical postgraduate colleges.
- National or government funding streams (such as the National Institute for Health Research in the UK, or the National Institute of Health in the USA).
- International public funding streams (such as the European research Council).
- Commercial (implant, pharmaceutical).
- University scholarships, studentships.
- Self pay.

Identify potential funding sources for applying to by searching the web, advert sites for research grants, speaking to peers or seniors who may have previously applied. In deciding where to apply you may consider:

- What is the remit of the funding stream? Does your proposal falls within that? What studies have been previously funded by that organisation?
- What grants are provided? Will it be enough? Are only large studies funded?
- How often are grants awarded?
- What is the application process (how many stages, average length of decision time)?

Applications for funding can be time consuming and often highly competitive. The following may help you prepare an application for a funding stream:

- Put together a well designed, scientifically sound study, justifying your methodology choices.
- Have a clearly written, well structured, succinct proposal that follows the rules and guidelines of the funding body.
- Clearly demonstrate what is the specific value of the proposed research and how does this fit within the remit of the funding stream? Whom will it benefit? How will it benefit? Why is it worth of funding?
- Use simple, plain language, with minimal technical terms – some reviewers may not be experts in the area of your research, but should still be able to understand what you propose.
- Demonstrate that what you propose is feasible and achievable. Anticipate potential issues such as low recruitment rates and specify how you plan to overcome this. Funders are looking for projects that can be delivered within the time and budget allocated.
- Try and put together a strong, reliable application team (team with strong track record with regards to previously obtaining funding, successfully completed funded projects, well published). If this is not possible remember that we all have to start somewhere. Justify the choice of each proposed team member, for their unique contribution.

- Involvement of patients or the general public in research design, is increasingly sought in funding applications. This may vary from the concept of idea, to study design, to patient information leaflet design, membership of study steering committees, dissemination of findings. State if such contribution has been made or is proposed. The questions that you may consider important in answering through research, may be different from those that patients consider important, hence their views are highly valued; you may consider important the exact position in which a bone fracture heals, but patients may consider more important the time they have to take off work whilst in plaster.
- If required give a lay summary of your study. Make it short, emphasising the aim and potential gains from this research.
- Give a summary of how your results will be disseminated.

Writing a Research Protocol

Write a research protocol, a predefined plan as to what you set out to do. Once this is done, it can be used as the basis for writing an Ethics committee application, funding application, institutional board application, and even later on, in writing up and publishing your research. This should contain sufficient information for some-one else to pick this research study up at any stage and follow what you set out to do. You may consider the following layout in writing a research protocol.

- Title
- Background

  - Rationale
  - What is known?
  - What is unknown?
  - What needs to be known?
  - Why is research necessary?
  - Who will benefit?
  - What will the specific benefits be?

- Aim – primary and other objectives
- Methods

  - Study design
  - Data collection
  - Data analysis

- Ethical considerations – local, regional, national application process. How often does ethics committee meet? When is the next application deadline?
- Resources needed
- Cost analysis
- Time scales for research progression and completion
- Dissemination of results (conferences/meetings, departmental, local, national, international, publications)

Audit

Audit is a process through which we aim to improve our practise, clinical or otherwise. In audit, we compare our current practise against an ideal practise, to allow us to identify deficiencies and areas for improvement (initial audit). We then introduce changes to address such deficiencies to try and meet that ideal. After introducing these changes and allowing time to be implemented and sustained, we re-examine our practise, to see whether we now meet the predefined ideal (re-audit). The audit loop (Fig. 7.3) is thus completed.

Standards of ideal practise may be set by the government, by healthcare organisations, by specialised medical bodies such as national medical or surgical associations, by patients or the general public, but some others, applicable to your direct practise, may be set by yourself.

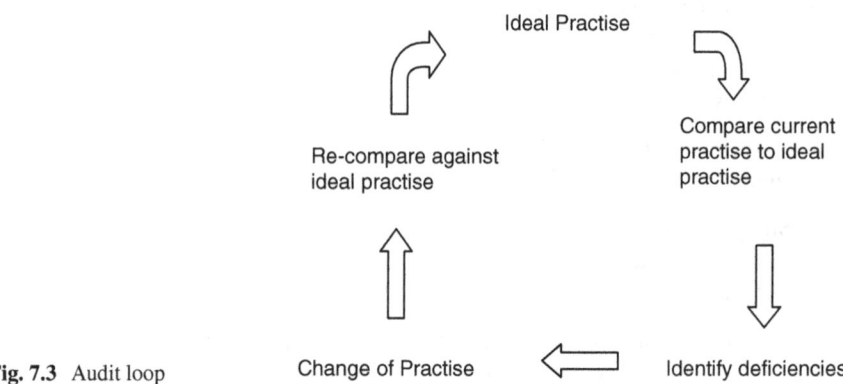

Fig. 7.3 Audit loop

Why Get Involved in Audit?

Audit acts as a mechanism of continuous service quality evaluation and improvement. It is the process that will help you evaluate and, if needed, further enhance your practise. Hence, the ability to identify areas that need auditing, and the ability to design and carry out an audit are important skills to develop. Getting involved in audits may help you develop such skills.

Audit allows you to quantify deficiencies and weaknesses of healthcare provision, and hence provides the justification for introducing changes. Such evidence may be essential in supporting the need for further resources, greater funding, better staffing, or new working patterns.

Audit is the process that may reassure you with quantified evidence, that your practise meets high quality standards. This can be used in personal evaluations, such as appraisals. Similarly, clinical audit is important for patients' and public reassurance. It gives confidence that individual doctors and healthcare organisations continuously assess their performance and strive for better care.

Carrying out an audit and implementing changes, may help you further develop your team working, leading, organisational and management skills.

Auditing may be an essential, government directed requirement of healthcare organisations, in healthcare systems of countries such as the UK [10].

For individual doctors getting involved in audits may help to strengthen your CV, and hence aid career progression. Audits are often considered essential or desirable, in job applications. Identifying an area to examine, leading and carrying out the primary audit, introducing changes, and finally leading and carrying out a re-audit, is considered the gold standard. Even if you can not carry out and complete the audit loop, carrying out an initial audit or a re-audit in isolation, may also be of value.

What Type of Audit to Do?

In your day to day clinical practise there are many areas that you may choose to audit. There are several types of audit:

- Audit of resources – availability and utilisation of resources such as staffing levels, skill mix, equipment, technology, space, time allocation, finances. Do we have the necessary critical care nurse numbers, midwives, junior doctors? Is there sufficient theatre time allocation for the number of surgeries we perform? Do we need more clinic space to reduce patient waiting times? Do we need more cubicles in the Emergency Department to avoid lengthy waits of patients in ambulances? Are resources used appropriately? Is there wastage of disposables in theatres, late starting and early finishing times of clinics, is specialised radiological imaging used responsibly, are costly non-evidence proven medications or surgical procedures utilised?
- Audit of process – Do our processes meet high standards? Such processes may include clinical assessment, communication with patients and staff, invasive surgical interventions, medical therapies, clinical tests, prescribing, documentation. Do we provide a smooth, fast medical service? What are the waiting times in clinics, Emergency Department, wait for surgery? Is there continuity of care? Do our patients receive essential prophylactic antibiotics or thrombo-prophylaxis? Do we make the correct diagnosis? Is the documentation in medical records eligible and thorough? Do we prescribe correctly? Do we follow institutional protocols and pathways?
- Audit of outcomes – Do we provide high quality care? What are our mortality and morbidity rates? Patient satisfaction and complaint rates? Patient reported outcomes? Hospitalisation length? Length of implant survival? Rates of stent occlusion? Rates of return to work, return to independent function, return to pre-injury activity levels? Do preventive measures achieve the desirable risk reduction?

You may audit the practise of one individual or a group of individuals, in one or multiple institutions. Audits may be local or more extensive, carried out at regional, national or international levels.

How to Identify an Area to Audit?

There are several ways in which you may identify a suitable area for auditing.

- Observation – You may notice an area in your daily clinical environment where things could be done better, and decide to assess it further. As a junior doctor you may spend more time in the ward than your seniors, and hence be in a central position to identify areas of potential improvement that your seniors may not be aware off. You may see an unusual complication and try and get to the bottom of why it happened. You may encounter the same issue over and over again, and decide to quantify the problem with the aim of initiating change.
- You may ask your seniors, colleagues, or juniors, for areas that they feel need looking into. Ask your patients as to what they feel needs improving or examined, as their perception of priorities may differ from yours.
- Your organisation may have specific audit priorities, audits that need to be carried out, as part of ensuring the provision of safe, high quality care. Your department's audit lead or audit department may advise you further.
- Complaints, near misses, or critical incidents, may indicate lapses in care, identifying areas to be further assessed.
- National/international published guidelines for clinical care, may give you ideas for audits to perform. Such guidelines may be produced by medical societies and government bodies. In the UK, the National Institute for health and Care Excellence publishes guidelines with regards the use of health technologies (such as medicines, treatments and procedures), clinical practice (appropriate management of certain diseases), health promotion, and social care. In the USA, the Agency for Healthcare Research and Quality provides medical guidelines. The Guidelines International Network also provides an international guideline library.

Audit Steps

Like in research, construct a plan, as how the audit (initial or re-audit) will be carried out, and write an audit protocol. This may be used in applications for institutional audit approvals and also for any funding applications.

You may consider the following generic layout for an audit protocol:

- Title.
- Background.

  - What practise is to be audited?
  - Why is an audit of this practise essential?
  - What is the current practise?
  - Guidelines against which the current practise will be audited.
  - Origin of these guidelines (international, national, systematic reviews, local).

- Audit design.

  - Define specific parameters/outcomes to be examined.
  - How will these be assessed and by whom?
  - Prospective/retrospective data collection.
  - Planned analysis of data.

- Users (such as patients, carers) involvement –from topic selection, to setting standards, implementing change.
- Audit team.
- Cost analysis, need for funding (institutional, government).
- Ethical considerations – patient and staff confidentiality, are data appropriate, data protection, length of data retention? Is any intervention above that used in normal clinical practise? Are patient surveys properly designed? What if you discover that harm has been done?
- Time scales for audit progression and completion.
- Dissemination of results (conferences/meetings, publications).
- Plans for introducing change if applicable – at individual, departmental, organisational level.
- Plans for sustaining change (regular monitoring).
- Plans for re-auditing (timeframe, audit team).

References

1. Oxford dictionaries. http://www.oxforddictionaries.com. Accessed 25 Sept 14.
2. National Institute for Clinical Excellence. Principles for best practice in clinical audit. Abingdon: Radcliffe Medical Press; 2002.
3. Famous Quotes at BrainyQuote. www.brainyquote.com. Accessed 23 Sept 14.
4. CareerYenta. http://careeryenta.wordpress.com. Accessed 26 Sept 14.
5. Sackett DL. Rules of evidence and clinical recommendations on the use of antithrombotic agents. Chest. 1989;95:2S–4.
6. Canadian task force on the periodic health examination. The periodic health examination. Can Med Assoc J. 1979;121:1193–254.
7. Sullivan D, Chung KC, Eaves 3rd FF, Rohrich RJ. The level of evidence pyramid: indicating levels of evidence in plastic and reconstructive surgery articles. Plast Reconstr Surg. 2011;128(1):311–4.
8. Goodreads. http://www.goodreads.com. Accessed 27 Sept 14.
9. World Medical Association. Declaration of Helsinki. http://www.wma.net. Accessed 27 Sept 14.
10. Research guidance. GMC. http://www.gmc-uk.org. Accessed 27 Sept 14.
11. Code of human research ethics. The British psychological society. http://www.bps.org.uk. Accessed 27 Sept 14.
12. McIntosh N, Bates P, Brykczynska G, Dunstan G, Goldman A, Harvey D, Larcher V, McCrae D, McKinnon A, Patton M, Saunders J, Shelley P. Guidelines for the ethical conduct of medical research involving children. Royal College of Paediatrics, child health: ethics advisory committee. Arch Dis Child. 2000;82(2):177–82.
13. Clinical audit. http://www.england.nhs.uk/ourwork/qual-clin-lead/clinaudit. Accessed on 27 Sept 14.

Chapter 8
Publishing and Presenting

Carrying out research or audit is essential in gathering new knowledge and information. However, such knowledge must be disseminated for the wider medical or scientific community to really learn and benefit from it. This chapter describes the Research and Audit Dissemination Cycles, and discusses how to publish your findings. The need for determination and perseverance is emphasised. This chapter finally concentrates on those skills required for successfully presenting your findings in scientific meetings, both through podium or poster presentations.

© Springer International Publishing Switzerland 2015   139
C. Panayiotou Charalambous, *Career Skills for Doctors*,
DOI 10.1007/978-3-319-13479-6_8

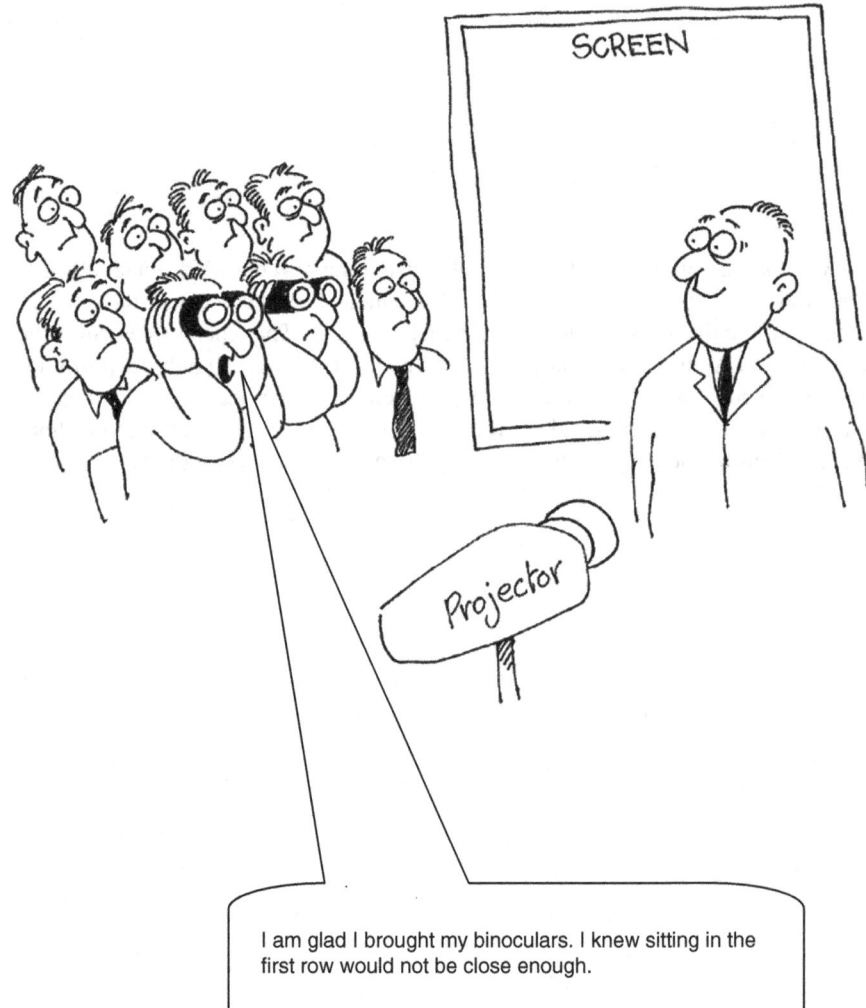

Research Dissemination

Dissemination of research findings could be described in terms of the Research Dissemination Cycle (Fig. 8.1), whereby research is carried out, and the results are then presented at local, national or international meetings. Research presented in such meetings may be subsequently published in a journal in abstract form, as part of an arrangement between the meeting organisers and the journal. The full research may also be submitted and published in a peer reviewed journal. Full publication further aids dissemination ensuring that generations to come will be able to access and benefit from that work. The published work may be read by other researchers, but also cited in future publications. Dissemination of research may provoke further research questions, leading to further research and re-starting of the cycle.

Unfortunately for much research the cycle is not completed, and often does not go beyond the research completion stage or presentation stage. A recent study showed that only about 37 % of presentations at the British Neurological Surgeons Society's meetings were eventually published as full articles [1]. This is consistent with a previous systematic review examining the fate of abstracts presented at biomedical meetings [2]. Some of the factors cited by authors for not proceeding to full publication are lack of time, low priority, anticipation of rejection and failure of the study to show positive results.

However, if you carried out a research project, collected the data, analysed your results, presented your findings and conclusions in meetings, then try and see it through and get it published. Why rush to starting a new research project if you have given up on publishing the last one? Getting an article published may show determination, and ability to see things through, rather than just taking on a task and leaving it half finished.

Even if unsuccessful in getting to present your research at a scientific meeting, it may still get published in full. Although presentation of research at a scientific meeting is strongly associated with subsequent full publication, it has been shown that about 30 % of research abstracts rejected from such meetings subsequently get published in full [2]. Acceptance in a meeting often depends on the popularity and size of the meeting, the number of podium or poster presentations allowed, and the number of submissions received, rather than simply on the quality or interest of your research.

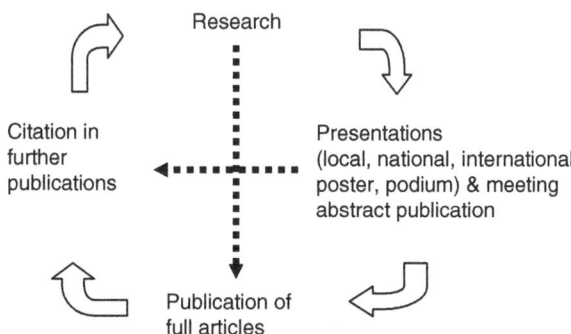

Fig. 8.1 The Research Dissemination Cycle. *Dashed arrows* indicate that stages of the cycle may be bypassed

Audit Dissemination

Like research, dissemination of audit findings is important to inform and educate stakeholders. An Audit Dissemination Cycle may thus be described. The main difference from the Research Dissemination Cycle is the strong local application of any findings which is highly relevant for many audits. However, presentation of findings through national or international meetings is also important, as other institutions or practitioners may learn from such experiences. Healthcare systems benefit through learning from each other's strengths or weaknesses. Some audits are performed at national or international level and hence they can be reported as such (Fig. 8.2).

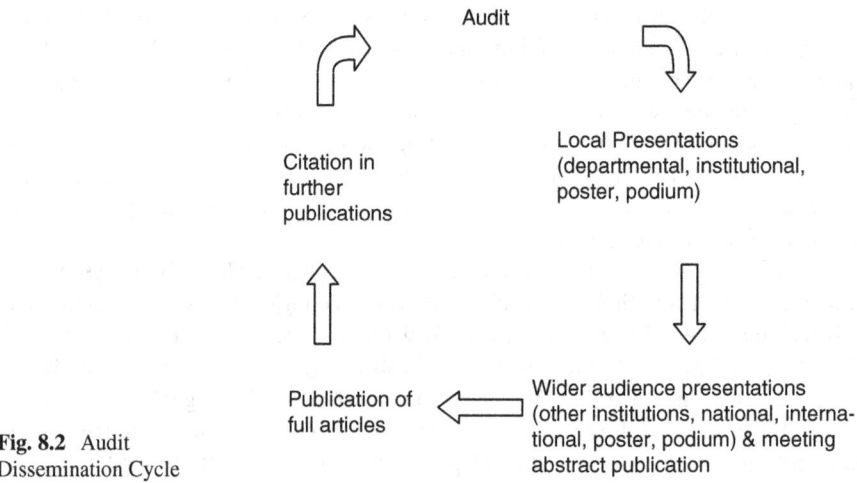

Fig. 8.2 Audit Dissemination Cycle

Publishing

You may be disappointed if you fail, but you are doomed if you don't try

Beverly Sills [3]

Carrying out research or audit and collecting data is only a small component of getting published. From data collection and analysis to full publication, there are several steps (Fig. 8.3). These steps include writing up an article, getting it checked and agreed by the various co-authors, and then submitting it for publication to a suitable journal.

A submitted article is usually initially checked by the administration of the journal, to confirm that is written according to the journal's instructions for authors with regards to, amongst others, layout and referencing. Its content is also initially assessed in house to determine whether it meets the scope of the journal, and hence whether it is suitable for publication in the journal.

Once these requirements are met, the article is usually sent out to two or more independent reviewers. The reviewers read the article, and advise on the potential suitability for publication. They take into account factors such as the originality, quality, relevance, importance and priority of the presented research study.

The journal editor then assesses these reviews, based on which a decision is made for the article to be rejected, accepted, or invited for revision and resubmission. If there is substantial disagreement between reviewers, the article may be sent out to another reviewer. Articles revised and resubmitted may have to be sent again to reviewers, depending on the level of revisions required (minor or major) or may simply be reviewed by the editor before a final decision is made. If finally accepted, the article will join the queue of articles awaiting publication in the journal. A fast track to publication may be available for some journals, where there is a need to disseminate a research message urgently. Prior to publication, the corresponding author is sent proofs of the article for final check and approval, where any typographical or grammatical changes may be made.

It can thus be seen that the review to acceptance and publication route is a lengthy, time consuming process. A recent study [4] looked at manuscripts published in the Australasian Medical Journal and found that the median duration of the review process was 74 days. Articles were returned to authors on average 1.7 times for revision. In about 36 % of papers instructions to authors were not adhered to, whilst about 30 % contained substantial grammatical errors. In 70 % of articles the invited reviewers did not return their reviews on time. A systematic review of the fate of abstracts presented at biomedical meetings and assessing the ones that finally got published in full, estimated that 27 % were published in full after two, 41 % after four, and 44 % after 6 years from presentation [2].

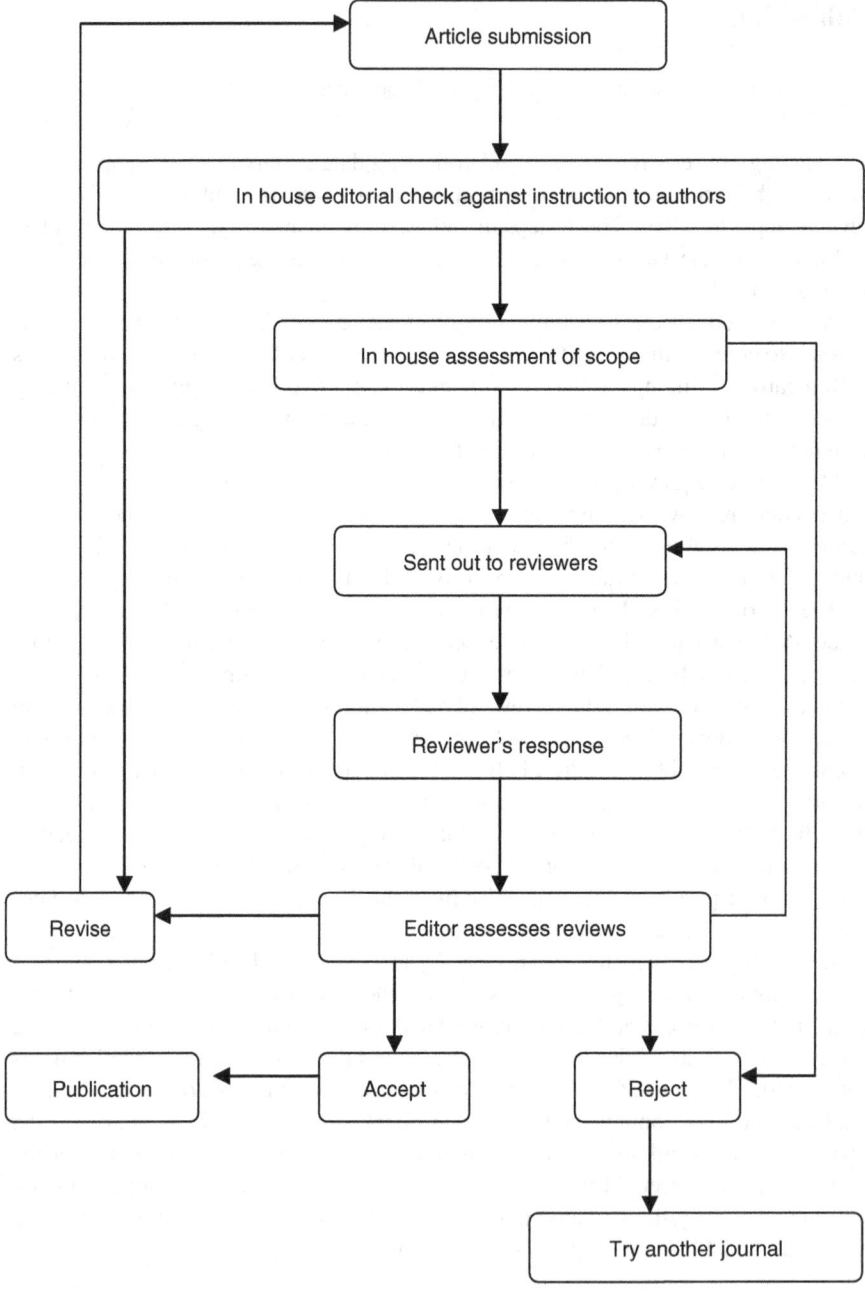

Fig. 8.3 The submission to publication process

Even though there are several steps in the submission to publication route there are only few, yet important steps, that you can directly influence to speed up the process:

- Submit your article promptly. Plan in advance, taking into account realistic timeframes.
- Ensure that your article adheres to the journal's instructions for authors. These may vary from journal to journal and the article must be adjusted according to the journal under consideration. Particular attention should be paid to style of referencing, format of figures and tables, use and explanation of abbreviations, layout of abstract and main text.
- Use simple, easily understood language, and avoid grammatical errors. If the journal language is not your first language, then get appropriate help.
- Make your article attractive to the reviewers.
- Choose the journal carefully, as further discussed below.
- Promptly re-submit, if asked to revise your article.
- If time goes and you have not heard back with regards your submission, a gentle email reminder, asking to trace your submission may speed up the process.

Which Journal to Publish In?

Once you write the article, the next decision is to which journal to get it submitted to be considered for publication. This will depend on the type of article and the quality of evidence the article provides. Given the length of the review process, journal choice is important in avoiding wasting time. In deciding which journal to submit to, you may consider:

- Discuss it with your seniors or colleagues.
- Does your article fall within the journal's scope and aims?
- Look at current and past issues of the journal. Does it publish articles similar to yours? If the journal has a policy against publishing systematic reviews should you be thinking of submitting one there?
- Reputation of the journal amongst researchers.
- Readership size and diversity of the journal.
- Target audience of your article – are you targeting a specialist or generalist group?
- Review time.
- Journal acceptance rate.
- Impact factor – this describes the average number of citations per article published in the journal in the previous 2 years. It is calculated by dividing the number of citations in the current year by the number of citable articles published in the last 2 years [5]. Although this is considered a crude measure of comparing quality of journals [6, 7], it is widely quoted. It does not take into account a journal's readership and the clinical impact published articles may have.

Do not be disappointed by rejection. An article may be rejected for several reasons and it does not necessarily mean that the quality of your research is poor. All that a rejection says, is that it was not judged suitable for publication by those specific peer reviewers and editor of a specific journal, at a particular time. It is possible for an article rejected by one journal to be subsequently successfully accepted in a more prestigious journal. Persevere and do not give up. Learn from any unsuccessful submissions, use any constructive feedback of reviewers to improve your article, and try again.

Publication Ethics

There are several ethical considerations in publishing. Some are plain obvious, some are more controversial:

Absolute nos

- Fabrication of results, methods – this is fraud.
- Misinterpretation of data, manipulation of images.
- Dual simultaneous submission – the same work can not be submitted to more than one journal simultaneously. This might increase your chances of a quicker publication, but is not acceptable.
- Duplicative publication – the same work can not be published in more than one journal.
- Plagiarism –this refers to using the work of others without appropriate referencing. The same applies to referring to own work, previously published elsewhere. Plagiarism check software can help you ensure this does not happen.
- Submission without prior agreement of all authors – get the final article version seen and agreed to by all authors, to avoid misunderstandings and subsequent need for retraction. Do not just assume that all authors will be glad to have their name on a published article.
- Fail to declare conflicts of interest – such as publishing an article reporting excellent results for a new medicine or implant, without declaring that you are a paid advisor for the company manufacturing the medicine or implant.
- Use of patient identifiable data without informed consent.

Controversial issues

- Authorship – It is essential to agree amongst collaborators of a research study, as to who will be the authors of any emerging articles, and what the order of authorship will be. The International Committee of Medical Journal Editors [8], gives guidance with regards authorship according to which authors should make substantial contribution in all the following domains:

  - Designing or running the research study
  - Preparing the article
  - Approving the final version of the article
  - Agreeing to be accountable for the work submitted

  However, even though, in an ideal situation all research members participate in all of the above domains, it is also possible that other workers, with particular expertise, are brought in at a later stage, as the need arises. If in doubt about authorship, clarify this with the editor of the journal you are submitting to, early on.

- Salami slicing –this refers to splitting data gathered from a single research project, and presenting and publishing those separately. This can lead to multiple smaller publications rather than a single wide publication. Such a practise is not appropriate simply for generating a greater publication volume. However, on occasions, it may be necessary to split data for presentation purposes. Such slicing may ensure that important messages are not lost or overseen as might happen in a wider publication [9–13]. If splitting data ensure this is clearly stated in your submitted article, and other publications related to the submission are clearly cited. If in doubt, discuss with journal editors prior to submission.

Stick to the rules, not only because it is the right approach, but also to avoid getting in trouble and putting your reputation at risk. If such practises are discovered journals may retract articles, ban authors from further submissions, and report authors to their institutions or professional regulatory bodies [14, 15].

Presenting Research in Meetings

Aim to present your research before it gets published. Many meetings will not accept presentations of research which has already been published in a journal. Presentation in meetings and conferences is important as:

- It is a vital stage of the Research Dissemination Cycle.
- Allows an initial presentation of your findings, giving you an indication as to how they are received by the wider research/scientific community.
- Questions raised in such meetings may help you prepare your article for full publication. Questions raised by the audience at such meetings may be similar to those raised later on by journal reviewers.
- Helps you improve your presentation skills.

Identify potential meetings early on. Application for presentation takes place in the form of abstract submission. Meetings open for abstract submission about a year in advance, with submission closing several months before the meeting. This allows reviews of the submitted abstracts, selection of those to be presented, notification of the authors, and finalisation of the program. Presentations may be in the form of podium or poster presentations. Some meetings require you to specify as to what you are submitting for, whilst others allow submission for either.

Identify potential meetings according to:

- Scope/aim of meeting.
- Target audience.
- Acceptance rate – size of meetings.
- Location of meetings – can you afford travelling to them?
- Regulations for submission – some meetings require the most senior author to be present if it gets accepted. Will that be possible?
- Have you presented elsewhere? – The same presentation can be submitted to multiple meetings, unless the meeting specifies otherwise.

Podium Presentations

Giving a scientific presentation is like telling a story, a tale story, a bedtime story. You set the context (background), you then describe what happened (methods), what was the outcome (results), and then you give the moral of the story (conclusions). However, unlike bedtime stories, you try to engage and enthusiase your audience, rather than talking them to sleep.

The ability to deliver a successful podium presentation is a skill to be developed and cultivated. The following may help you in this:

- Use a short, catchy title for your presentation.
- Keep your presentation simple, use plain language, keep it to the level of your audience.
- Succinct – many of us have a tendency to give all facts, make sure we did not leave anything behind. However, even though you may have spent 3 years on your research project, hove tons of results and lots of conclusions, it would be unrealistic to try and fit all that in a 5 or 10 min presentation. Concentrate on the most important aspect of your work, or the part relevant to the meeting and simply present that.
- Slides:

  - Be minimalistic
  - Avoid slide overcrowding
  - Be consistent on font type and size
  - Ensure font size can be clearly read from the back of the room
  - Choose eye friendly background and text colours
  - Use contrast between text and background colour

- Graphs:

  - Keep graphs simple
  - Well labelled
  - Use easily read axes

  When you show a slide with a graph pause momentarily, and give your audience time to digest it. Point to the axes and demonstrate what they stand for.
- Avoid videos that may not run on the day.
- Take backups of your talk. Email your presentation to yourself as a backup too.
- Dress for the occasion.
- Know your equipment – microphone, pointer, projector control (how can you move to next slide or go back one).
- Get to the venue early, dry run your presentation, ensure that the format of your slide does not change due to incompatible software.
- Body language is important. Look confident, upright posture.
- Use confident strong voice.
- Prior to starting your talk, thank the chair person. The chair person will usually introduce you to the audience, and hence further verbal introduction of your self is not essential.

- Look at your audience. Rather than looking to the ceiling or the floor look at audience members.
- Speak slowly enough to be understood and be followed, but fast enough to keep your audience engaged.
- Use pointers with caution. Pointing to every word as you read it adds nothing. Use pointers to highlight facts, explain graphs, and demonstrate relevant parts of figures or pictures.
- At the beginning of your talk, as you put up your first slide, look at the screen, and ensure the slide has appeared on the screen. Do not go half way through your talk, until you realise there is a problem with the projector and slides are not showing up.
- Watch your pace. Avoid being too slow or too fast. Use the time needed to pass the message of each slide. The pace may vary from slide to slide. Spend longer on those slides that may be more difficult to understand, less on the straightforward ones. Spend more time on slides that are vital in communicating your overall message.
- Stick to the time – you really do not want the chairman of the meeting to stop you half way through. Imagine a day program of 10 min talks, equal to 42 talks in total. If each presenter overruns by 2 min, by the end of the day you will be running 1.5 h behind.
- Avoid reading your slides. Your audience, in most cases at least, should be able to read. Talk about your slides in a different way. After all, if all you are doing is reading your slides, you could have posted them to the audience with no need to turn up.
- Avoid speaking from notes. It may be better to say less, but appear as if words come from your heart, rather than say lots from paper sheets. It gives confidence to the listener that you know what you are talking about, and that what you are telling them is second nature to you. After all you did the research hence you should be able to talk about it.
- Have confidence and passion.
- Enjoy the talk. You are fortunate enough to have your presentation accepted and your research to be presented. It is an opportunity to tell others about what you have achieved, an opportunity to disseminate your research.
- Practise your presentation- if you are due to present in a national conference, try and present your findings to your department or other peers beforehand. Apart from allowing practise of all the skills described above, such a dry run is likely to raise questions similar to those asked later by the conference audience.
- Anticipate questions and practise answers.

Poster Presentations

Posters may be in the form of printed paper or electronic format. Printed posters are put on display on walls and boards in the conference venue. Electronic posters may be in the form of slides, such as power-point, and are viewed in computers or tablets in the venue. Attendants walk by and view the posters. You may be required to formally attend some of these viewing sessions, where you stand by your poster and answer questions.

In preparing a poster the first step is to ask the meeting organisers for their poster preparation guidelines. Closely follow those guidelines with regards to poster size, format, layout, and content presentation. Nevertheless, whatever the meeting's regulations, there are several steps that you can take to ensure that your poster is well presented, clearly transmits the necessary message, attracts attention, and is hence read by a wide audience.

A poster is like a painting. Art galleries have numerous paintings on display, yet only a few of these may attract enough attention of walkers by, to make them stop and devote time to view and admire them. The following may improve the appeal of your poster:

- Short catching title.
- Plain background.
- Minimal text, text boxes.
- Good font size, easy to read.
- Contrast between text and background colour.
- Lots of pictures, graphs, figures.
- High quality illustrations.
- Simple layout.
- Clear aim and conclusion.
- Succinct methods section.

References

1. Jamjoom AA, Hughes MA, Chuen CK, Hammersley RL, Fouyas IP. Publication fate of abstracts presented at Society of British Neurological Surgeons meetings. Br J Neurosurg. 2014.
2. von Elm E, Costanza MC, Walder B, Tramèr MR. More insight into the fate of biomedical meeting abstracts: a systematic review. BMC Med Res Methodol. 2003;3:12.
3. Goodreads. http://www.goodreads.com. Accessed on 25 Sept 2014.
4. Cornelius JL. Reviewing the review process: identifying sources of delay. Australas Med J. 2012;5(1):26–9.
5. Amin M, Mabe M. Impact factors: use and abuse. Perspect Publ. 2001;1:1–6.
6. Kurmis AP. Understanding the limitations of the journal impact factor. J Bone Joint Surg Am. 2003;85-A(12):2449–54.
7. Haddad FS. The impact factor: yesterday's metric? Bone Joint J. 2014;96-B(3):289–90.
8. International Committee of Medical Journal Editors. Defining the role of authors and contributors. http://www.icmje.org. Accessed on 23 Sept 2014.
9. Mojon-Azzi SM, Mojon DS. Scientific misconduct: from salami slicing to data fabrication. Ophthalmic Res. 2004;36(1):1–3.
10. Karlsson J, Beaufils P. Legitimate division of large data sets, salami slicing and dual publication, where does a fraud begin? Knee Surg Sports Traumatol Arthrosc. 2013;21(4):751–2.
11. Jackson D, Walter G, Daly J, Cleary M. Editorial: multiple outputs from single studies: acceptable division of findings vs. 'salami' slicing. J Clin Nurs. 2014;23(1–2):1–2.
12. Klein AA, Pozniak A, Pandit JJ. Salami slicing or living off the fat? Justifying multiple publications from a single HIV dataset. Anaesthesia. 2014;69(3):195–8.
13. Norman G. Data dredging, salami-slicing, and other successful strategies to ensure rejection: twelve tips on how to not get your paper published. Adv Health Sci Educ Theory Pract. 2014;19(1):1–5.
14. Steen RG. Retractions in the scientific literature: is the incidence of research fraud increasing? J Med Ethics. 2011;37(4):249–53.
15. Fang FC, Steen RG, Casadevall A. Misconduct accounts for the majority of retracted scientific publications. Proc Natl Acad Sci U S A. 2012;109(42):17028–33.

Chapter 9
Managing and Leading

Managing and leading often form an integral part of a doctor's daily work life. Apart from managing yourself, your own time and affairs, you may get involved in managing others, your team, your clinic, your department, your hospital or institution. You may manage a process, a project, the rota, the teaching program, the theatre list allocation. You may manage a conflict, a meeting, or manage change.

You may be called upon not just to follow, but also lead. You may lead your juniors, your team, your colleagues, your department, your organisation. You may lead the resuscitation team, the theatre operating team, the clinic team, the discharge multidisciplinary team.

There are certain skills that may help in such challenging roles. Managing and leading require good communication and interpersonal skills. This chapter aims at describing these skills that you may try to develop early on.

At the same time, you may find yourself on the receiving end of management. Even as part of a formal managerial role you may have to deal with more senior managers. The ability to deal effectively with management, in a constructive and mutually respective manner, is an additional valuable skill to acquire.

© Springer International Publishing Switzerland 2015
C. Panayiotou Charalambous, *Career Skills for Doctors*,
DOI 10.1007/978-3-319-13479-6_9

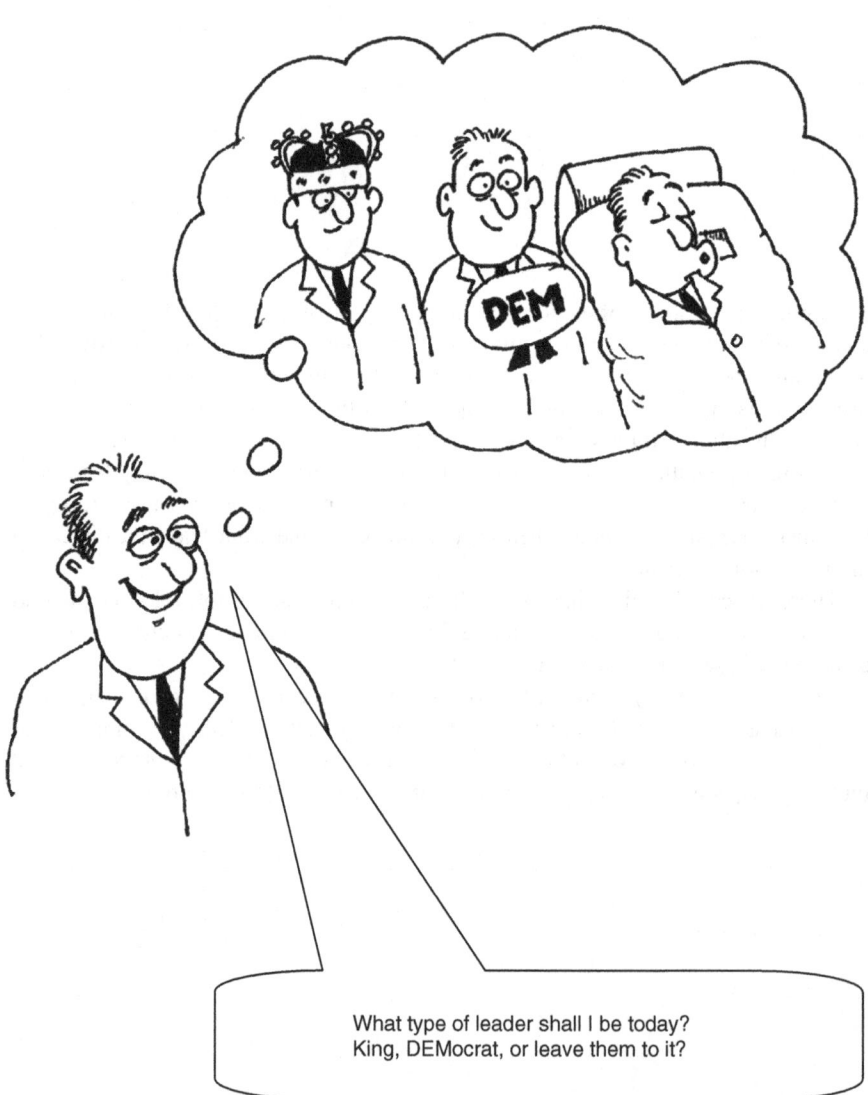

Inter-personal Skills

Governing a great nation is like cooking a small fish – too much handling will spoil it
Lao-tzu [1]

Whether managing or leading, certain skills are essential. Unlike a few lucky ones, many of us are not born natural managers or leaders, but these roles need to be cultivated and developed. Management and leadership involves closely working with people, and certain skills are essential in such interpersonal relationships.

Different styles of management/leadership have been described [2, 3] but three well known ones are:

1. Authoritative – leader decides and followers do.
2. Democratic – leader and followers share decision making.
3. Laissez-faire – leader delegates the tasks to the followers, who are allowed to take control and influence how things are done.

The type of management/leadership you choose is likely to be influenced by your status, your personality, followers, and tasks to be accomplished. The style chosen does not have to be rigid and may vary according to the situation, individuals or processes you are dealing with. The decision as to what type of leader to be is yours, but you may consider the following in trying to develop your managerial and leadership skills:

Lead by Example

Lead by example and inspire others. Encouraging others to do as you do is more effective than simply asking them to do as you say. If you are the first to turn up to the ward, if you are hands on and do not shy off seeing patients in clinic, if you rush to help colleagues when in need, if you do not hesitate to stand up and take responsibility for your actions, if you easily acknowledge when things have gone wrong, if all your actions have in heart the good of patients and your organisation, others may be inspired and follow promptly.

Involve

As a doctor, you are likely to be managing other highly motivated individuals, such as doctors or other healthcare workers. These, alongside you, are striving for providing the best of care. Consult them for their opinions and listen actively to what they have to say. Involve all those you manage, all those you lead. Hear the arguments, encourage discussions. Do not use listening as a mere exercise, but as an improvement process. Decisions taken by consensus or majority, through constructive discussions, may be more likely to be respected and followed.

Be Straight

Be honest, direct, and straight, in trying to pass a message across, or convince others. Attempts to pass a policy on the side may simply cause loss of trust and confidence, when the whole picture is established. Even if you have to give awkward news, be honest, direct and truthful.

Respect Your Followers

Respect your followers. Avoid talking bad about your followers, in front of others. This will encourage trust, and your followers will know that you will not fail them.

Support

Support and stand by those you manage or lead at the time of need. It may be your juniors have just started and are trying to find their feet. It maybe, a colleague is going through difficult times at home, and needs to take time off at short notice. This is the time to stand by them, help, and support them.

Have a Vision

Have a clear vision as to what you are trying to achieve and work for it. Communicate this to your followers. Give a clear goal to work towards.

Enable

Trust your team. If they are safe, keen, competent and skilled, let them get on with it. You do not have to micromanage, check and control all they do.

Give Clear Instructions

Give clear instructions so that others can understand easily and follow. You may communicate your reasoning and your thinking, but aim to give a clear direction, explicit details of what has to be done, and how it is to be achieved.

Give an Answer Rather than Options

As a doctor you may be seen as a leading figure, both by medical but also other healthcare professionals who will come to you for answers. Give them what they ask for, rather than a list for options to choose from.

Appreciate the Diversity of Those You Manage or Lead

Appreciate that your followers may have different priorities, personal beliefs, different backgrounds, previous experiences. The world is a global village. Your followers may originate from different ethnicities, or cultures. It is unlikely that one approach, one solution will fit all situations or all individuals.

Rely on Systems, Not Just Individuals

Set up well structured, functioning, self relying systems, policies, protocols and pathways, rather than just relying on individuals doing their best. People may move on, progress in their career or retire, their duties may change, may go off sick, may be on leave, may be off shift. Aim for systems, procedures, and protocols that are easy to grasp, simple to understand, and plain to follow through. Some of the staff, such as those in training posts, may rotate regularly, spending only a short time in your team, department, or institution. Well structured systems should ensure that new starters settle in quickly, fit in their new role, and service lapses and interruptions are kept to a minimum.

See the Big Picture

Concentrate on the details, but also see the big picture. Do not lose sight of the forest for the trees. The Seven S model, may put a structure, into how you assess the resources available within your team, organisation or department. It may help you determine as to whether all resources are working towards achieving the overall goal, working in line with the overall vision [4]. The seven S model stands for:

S-tructure
S-trategy
S-ystems
S-taff
S-kills
S-tyle
S-uper ordinate goal

Be Lean

As a manager or leader you may face longstanding procedures or processes which may not be cost or time effective. Challenge these, aim to improve efficiency, and maximise value. Lean principles were initially derived from the car manufacturer Toyota, but have widely been adopted in health care [5, 6]. Lean principles put the provision of high quality service (or care) to the customer (or in a healthcare setting the patient) central to the organisation's aim. Processes that work towards providing that high quality service are identified, enhanced and smoothed out, whilst any unnecessary steps or processes (waste) are eliminated. Reducing low yield steps and processes may thus reduce the time and resources needed for providing high quality care [7–9].

Aim for Big Wins

Aim to solve those problems, and tackle those challenges, that can make a substantial difference, and achieve huge improvements. According to the Pareto principle (80–20 rule), 80 % of problems may be caused by 20 % of causes. Vilfredo Pareto was an Italian economist early in the 1900s who noticed that 80 % of land in Italy was held by 20 % of the population. Interestingly, he then went on to notice that 20 % of pea pods in his garden gave 80 % of all peas. Joseph Juran, an engineer, reported that this principle also applied to engineer defects (20 % of defects causing 80 % of problems), and named this the Pareto principle [10–15]. This principle has since been applied to other settings. Even though the exact application of this in healthcare remains to be established [16], it helps to remind that some problems may cause more trouble than others and tackling those can have a much greater effect. It does not mean ignoring the remaining 80 % of causes, but prioritising according to potential influence and importance.

Use Targets Wisely

Talent hits a target no one else can hit; Genius hits a target no one else can see
Arthur Schopenhauer [1]

Targets are often set as a guide of what we are aiming to achieve. When applied correctly, targets aim to bring forwards changes in service provision, and work patterns, to improve care quality. They may be self imposed, set by your organisation, the government. Understand what targets aim to achieve, and work towards that. Use the target as a means of improving your service, as an empowering tool for driving the essential care improvement, rather than altering your service to improve your target performance.

In the National Health System of the UK, multiple health care targets were introduced by the government. These included a 4 h rule for either admission or discharge from the Emergency Department, an 18 week target to reduce surgical waiting lists, 2 day target within which patients should be able to see their general practitioner [17].

Meeting such targets would ensure that patients do not wait long for a decision in the Emergency Department, have easy access to their family doctor, and do not face unnecessary delays in having elective surgery. Keeping patients in ambulances to stop the Emergency Department clock start ticking, admitting patients unnecessarily, discharging patients too early, offering patients surgery on days or at venues that they are unlikely to meet, or focusing on patients who have not missed the target at the expense of those that missed the target, is not a wise or ethically correct way of target use [18–21].

Targets are important in setting a well defined structure as to what you are working to, hence make the most of them. But do not miss the point trying to meet the target. Much of Medicine, much of the service you provide, much of what you do, day in and day out, may not be easily measured or quantified. Do not overlook quality, or true caring, for running after a target.

Value Productivity Rather than Time

Stressing output is the key to improving productivity, while looking to increase activity can result in just the opposite

Paul Gauguin [1]

Often what counts more, is not how much time or effort goes into achieving a goal, but the achievement of the goal per se. Output may be more important than input. This may be a metric in evaluating people or processes you manage or lead.

Output rather than input, may apply not only to individuals but also to systems of whole countries or huge organisations. Figures from the Organisation for Economic Co-operation and Development suggest that in 2013 the average Greek worker clocked 2,036 h whereas the average German worker only about 1,387 h [22]. Yet the economy of Germany has recently been thriving, whilst that of Greece has gone through substantial turmoil. Many successful organisations have moved from counting minutes of their employees to assessing their output. The Results Only Work Environment (ROWE) refers to a management approach where performance and results, rather than mere presence, is rewarded [23]. ROWE was initially introduced at the electrical retailer Best Buy, to increase productivity, and was adopted by several institutions since then, including GAP, the clothing retailer. Staff were given the freedom to work whenever they want and wherever they want, as long as the work gets done. Not all activities in healthcare can be arranged like that, yet some, like administrative or teaching tasks may be.

Consider judging others based on their achievements, rather than the time they put in. It maybe your junior can finish the ward work quickly and then relax in the coffee shop. It maybe a colleague is a fast surgeon and can finish the operating list quickly. It maybe a colleague can evaluate patients much more quickly in clinic and hence finish early. Consider concentrating on results, not the clock.

In healthcare, remuneration by results has been questioned, but this may be due to the metrics used. If all that is counted is the number of patients one assesses, or the number of operations one performs, without taking into account the outcomes achieved, or the complexity of cases dealt with, then obviously the process may be flawed.

Be Flexible and Accommodative

Nothing is softer or more flexible than water, yet nothing can resist it

Lao Tzu [1]

As a leader or manager it is essential to bring everyone on board, to motivate your followers. Being flexible and accommodative may help you do so. Appreciate that the values and requirements of one team member may be different from those of others. Treat everyone as an individual and try to accommodate their specific needs. If you can accommodate their individual needs without compromising the overall service, then try and do so, as that may further motivate them and encourage them to give their best self.

- It maybe that one junior wants to work with a specific team, to improve their surgical skills in a particular procedure.
- It maybe that your junior wants to come in early and finish early, to pick the kids from school.
- It maybe that a junior wants to have their holidays just before their upcoming exam, for better preparation.
- It maybe a colleague wants to take time off clinical work, to get that research project started.

Do not assume that all your followers are guided by the same motives, do not assume that your followers' motives are the same as yours. Something looking trivial to you may be highly important to others. Something that makes you tick may be of low importance to your followers. It has been shown that once people get enough food on the table, other factors may become important for job satisfaction. Daniel Pink in his book "Drive: the surprising truth about what motivates us"[24] dismisses the traditional models of motivation based on monetary rewards or fear of punishment, and describes three other elements as important in motivating individuals to give their best self at work. Quoting research done at the Massachusetts Institute of Technology, USA, Pink proposes that for complex, mind engaging activities, the three most important motivators are:

- Autonomy.
- Mastery.
- Purpose.

Indeed, you may recognise that the freedom to innovate and develop one's own work, the drive to excel professionally, and the feeling of making a real contribution, is the driver and real motivators for many healthcare workers in your workplace.

Along similar lines, more than half a century earlier, Abaraham Maslow, proposed a hierarchy of needs, in his paper "A theory of human Motivation" [25]. This is an idea widely depicted to today as Maslow's pyramid (Fig. 9.1). In this pyramid the most physiological basic needs are placed at the bottom, which once met, higher levels of needs are desired. It reminds that once there is enough bread on the table, then security, friendships, respect, and a drive to achieving one's full potential may become more important aspirations.

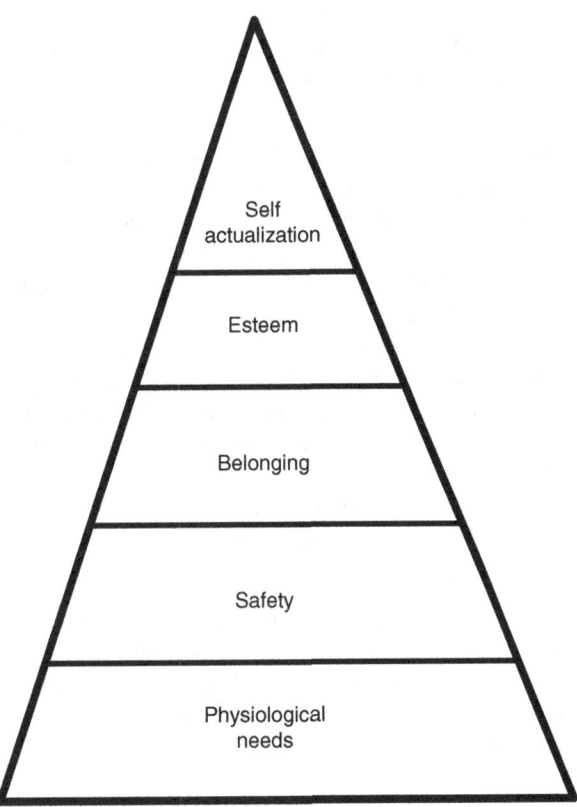

Fig. 9.1 Maslow's pyramid of hierarchy of needs (Based on Maslow [25])

Delegate

> Few things can help an individual more than to place responsibility on him, and to let him know that you trust him
>
> Booker Washington [10]

Delegation is not only important when it comes to sharing individual work, but is also an important skill of management. You may delegate the roles in your team, department or institution, the various roles in an audit or research project, the roles in an educational program. The skill is to delegate to those that will stand up to the challenge and will successfully complete the task. You may look for the 5As in deciding whom to delegate specific roles:

A-ble. Chose someone who has the ability, knowledge, skills, qualifications to fulfil the assigned task. Some of us may be excellent communicators, some are negotiators, some have an academic incline, some shine technically. Choose the most able person according to the task required.

A-uthorised. Choose someone who has the stature or authority to complete the role. This may be based on the chosen's seniority, experience, status, position, reputation, influence.

A-vid. Choose someone who is keen, enthusiastic on taking on the task. A genuine interest in the proposed task may encourage one giving best self. Not all tasks can be equally exciting and inspiring. Not all tasks will attract someone's attention, and on occasions you may have to allocate tasks to those who are not keen to take them on.

A-ttested – someone reliable, with a track record of delivering.

A-ccountable – someone who can take responsibility for the successful completion of the task.

Once you delegate, trust those taking on the task to see it through. Offer access, support, guidance and assistance, but have the confidence in those you chose. Delegating tasks, but still running the show, may defeat the purpose. The aim is not simply to have an additional pair of hands, but share development and responsibility.

Managing a Meeting

If they can't start a meeting without you, well, that's a meeting worth going to, isn't it? And that's the only kind of meeting you should ever concern yourselves with

George Huang [26]

As a doctor you may have to manage or lead a meeting, a meeting of your colleagues or team, to discuss business matters, to set policies and direction. Leading a meeting is an important skill to develop, and you may consider the following:

- Give ample notice about the meeting taking place.
- Send out, well in advance, documents relevant to the meeting, to allow participants to fully examine them.
- Invite only those relevant to the agenda and who will have a direct contribution to make. Attendants are not there for making up the numbers, but for making a real contribution.
- Avoid distractions, mobile phones, bleeps. Ask attendants to address these.
- Have a clear agenda for the meeting.
- Have a clear target for each agenda item (discuss or make decision) and aim to achieve that.
- Be clear who will deal with each item.
- Set realistic time frame, for each item, and stick to it. You do not want participants leaving halfway through.
- Decide how decisions will be made. If this is by majority, how many attendants are required?
- Keep clear records (minutes) of what is said at the meeting.
- Following the meeting, check the accuracy of the minutes with everyone who attended.
- Choose a place where interruptions are unlikely. A note on the door or a locked door may help, if you can not find a location away from the floor.
- Respect all those attending, their views and opinions, the time they put in attending the meeting. Give them the chance to speak and listen wisely. For a meeting to happen, for you to lead, others must turn up.

Managing Change

The only way to make sense out of change is to plunge into it, move with it, and join the dance

Alan Watts [1]

Healthcare is a dynamic environment. Changes often have to be introduced and you may find your self in a position where you have to manage and lead such changes; the introduction of a new rota, new working patterns, new team structures, new letter dictation system, new patients' charts recording system, departments merging, services tailored down or expanded. Managing change is a challenging task, often due to the anxiety of the unknown.

In introducing change, try to demonstrate clearly the need for change (Why change), the destination you are aiming to reach (Where), and the process (Way) by which this will be achieved (Fig. 9.2).

Recall the last time a change in practise was thrust upon you. You might have been told that this is how things should now be done, or told off for not doing them, without having been informed of the change in the first place. How engaged did that make you? How keen did that make you in joining and following the new practise?

In managing change consider the following:

- Engage others in understanding the need of change. If you get them on board as to why change is needed, it is more likely that you will achieve cooperation. Even if you can not engage all, the more the better. Jo Owen in his book "How to

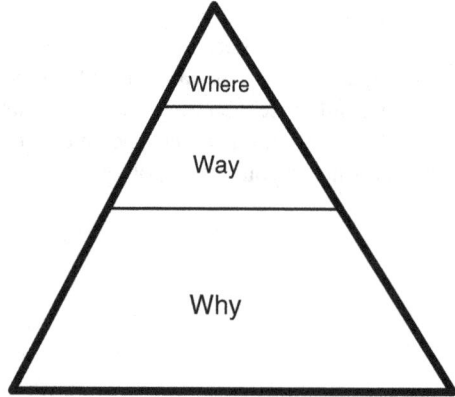

Fig. 9.2 The change pyramid – the base (or foundation) of achieving change is often to demonstrate the need for it. The destination must be clearly defined, and the way to it clearly characterised

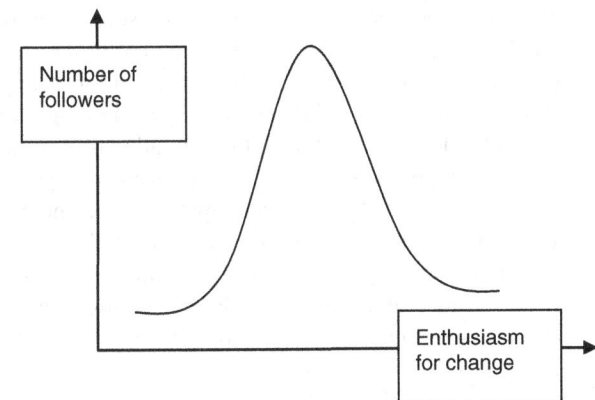

Fig. 9.3 Distribution of enthusiasm for change amongst potential followers (Adapted from Owen [27])

lead" [27], describes a bell shaped distribution of enthusiasm amongst those involved in a change process (Fig. 9.3), and argues that the main aim is to engage the main mass, rather than the few who regularly provide opposition. To engage this mass and gain core support, communicating the need for change and providing constant progress information are crucial.

- Explain to all, what is in it for them. The more winners out of a change, the more widespread its acceptance is likely to be.
- Consult wisely. Listen to what others have to say, and where possible follow their advice. If you achieve consensus, or reach an acceptable middle ground, it may be more likely for change to work.
- Demonstrate clearly the pathway to change. How will it be achieved, timescales, reviews of process. Reduce uncertainty to the minimum possible. Reduce fears, concerns and anxieties, through an open and transparent process.
- Be honest, do not overplay the situation, explain the limitations of any new undertaking, and acknowledge anticipated problems.
- Following introduction of the change, have regular reviews, to assess progress.
- Be flexible. If things do not work out as initially planned be prepared to adjust the course.
- Be aware that an early enthusiasm may wear off, and at the first difficulties doubts may mount. Keep the direction and drive.
- Communicate – maintain regular effective communication as to the progress, difficulties, and diversions from the original plan.
- Collect evidence – collect data to assess progress. Share these with all those involved.
- Take into account the expected responses when encountering change. Elizabeth Kubler-Ross, an American psychiatrist, developed in the 1960s [28] a model to explain five stages of the grieving process of terminally ill patients learning their

diagnosis. These stages may be also be seen in individuals undergoing major change [29] and has led to the development of the change curve, to help predict performance following the announcement of change [30]. The five stages (Fig. 9.4) are shock and denial, anger, bargaining, depression, and acceptance. Some individuals may not go through all stages or in that particular sequence. However, appreciating that those involved may go through these stages, may help you understand what to anticipate and thus help them through. The change curve helps to realise that after some initial enthusiasm, as the reality sinks in and despair predominates, there may be a time of real opposition to the occurring change. Anticipating this, and communicating to those involved, may help you push through, rather than giving up [29].

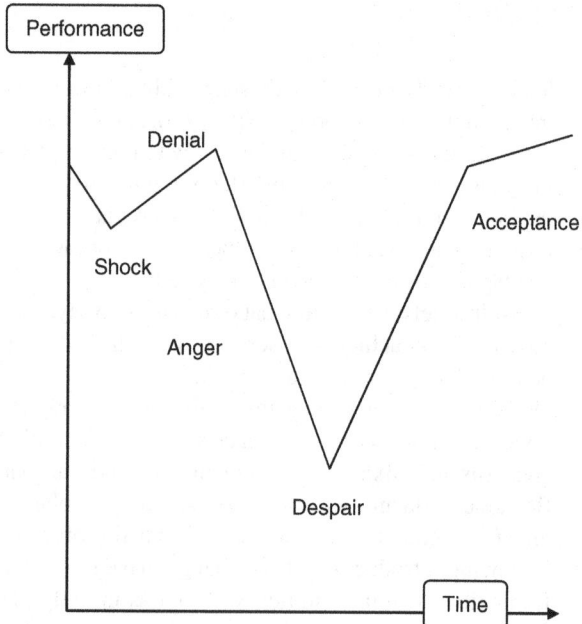

Fig. 9.4 The change curve (Adapted from The Change Curve, University of Exeter [30])

Managing a Project

The only way to do great work is to love what you do

Steve Jobs [1]

There may be times when you take on a project, and you have to see it through. It is likely that implementation does not rely solely on your input but needs the contribution and participation of others. In taking on and managing a project consider the following:

- Have a clear definition and understanding of what the project involves. Break it down into small parts to get a better grasp of what is required.
- Time management. Have clear starting and finishing targets, with milestone dates in between.
- Have a structured way of assessing or tackling a proposed project, rather than just jumping straight in. Different assessment systems have been used but PEST [31] and SWOT [32] may be useful.

PEST analysis refers to taking into account the

P-olitical
E-conomic
S-ocial
T-echnological

factors that may influence your endeavour. Inclusion of environmental, legal, ethical, and demographic factors have also been added, giving a wide range of acronyms.

SWOT analysis involves assessing the new project with regards its:

S-trengths – advantages over others
W-eaknesses – weaknesses compared to others
O-pportunities – what could the opportunities be?
T-hreats – what could cause trouble?

- Determine what resources you will need. Are these available? Can they be obtained? Do you have to put other tasks on the side to take this on?
- Set achievable, realistic, but also testing deadlines.

Managing Crises

Close scrutiny will show that most 'crisis situations' are opportunities to either advance, or
stay where you are

Maxwell Maltz [1]

As a doctor, you are likely to face crises, in direct clinical care or otherwise. A patient may crash in the ward or start bleeding profusely in the middle of surgery. The Emergency Department may be overwhelmed following a bus crash, or the medical ward may be overwhelmed following a flu outbreak. Your department may be short staffed due to skill shortage and poor recruitment. The financial situation may be dire, close to the brink of closing wards, and losing services.

How to deal with a crisis may require knowledge, technical skills, foresight and advanced preparation. Institutional patient pathways or protocols may already be in place to deal with anticipated crises. It is necessary to ensure you are familiar with these. However, in times of crises a set of appropriate behaviours is also essential. In dealing with crises consider:

- Keep your composure.
- Appear and sound confident – think of the pilot's voice, last time you went through a bad bout of turbulence.
- Show that you are in control. Others may be looking to you for leadership, and direction. If you can not be in control or lead, then let someone else take over.
- Assertive communication – ensure that you are listened to and everyone is focussed on the task.
- Delegate, give clear instructions and roles to all those involved.
- Communicate – explain what the plan is, give a running commentary, so that all can recognise you are on top of things.
- This is not the time to shout, complain, assign blame. Reflection may be necessary, but at a later stage.
- Anticipate crises, and practise how you would behave, if found in the middle of one. Simulate for crises. Practise talking or giving instructions as if you are under pressure.

Managing Conflict

Conflict is very much a state of mind. If you're not in that state of mind, it doesn't bother you
                                                                          Yotam Ottolenghi [1]

Conflict may be defined as a "disagreement within oneself or between people that causes harm or has the potential to cause harm" [33]. As a doctor, you may find yourself managing conflict. This maybe with an upset patient, an angry colleague or other staff. It may be your own or someone else's conflict. It maybe that your juniors can not get on with each other, that a junior is struggling with a nurse in the ward, or that two colleagues keep arguing.

You may approach conflict in a three step way (de-escalation triangle) whereby you firstly try to calm the tense situation, followed by finding out what the issues are, and then negotiating/working towards a solution [26]. However, beware that this may be an evolving process and you may have to move back and forth between steps. You may be negotiating but tempers may rise again. You may be negotiating only to find out that there are still facts to learn (Fig. 9.5). In dealing with conflict, consider that give and take is part of professional life. Try and find a mid-solution, if that is possible. Each of the three steps of conflict management requires certain approaches:

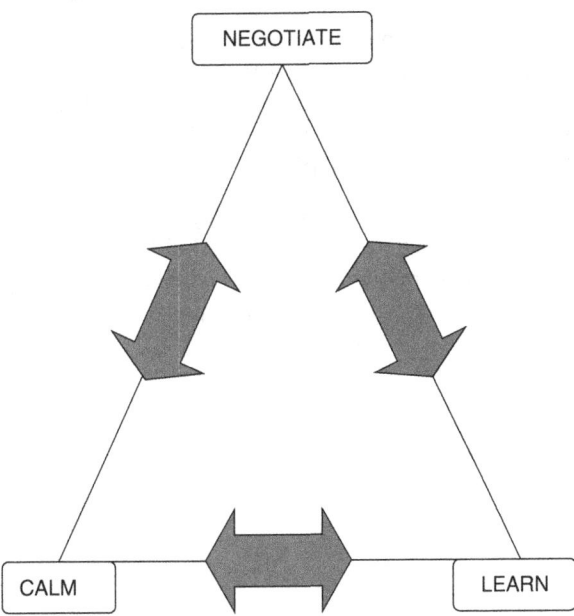

Fig. 9.5 The de-escalation triangle for conflict management

Calm:	de-escalate the situation
	change environment to help tempers settle
	acknowledge the frustration
	empathise
	sympathise
Learn:	stop and listen.
	find what the issues are
	why is the other party upset?
	hear the other side of the story
Negotiate:	What does the other party want?
	What are you after?
	What can you give?
	What is essential to take?
	Can an acceptable solution be reached?

A commonly used tool for assessing self awareness, the Thomas-Kilmann Conflict Mode Instrument [34], describes five ways of dealing with conflict:

Competing – one puts self over others.
Collaborating – work together for a solution.
Compromising – one considers both self and others.
Avoiding – one ignores self and others.
Accommodating – one puts others over self.

Which approach you take may depend on the situation, on what the issue is, and how much it matters to you. It is a skill to be able to pick your fights carefully, to decide which are worth fighting, and which ones are to be ignored. Decide when you have to win, when you can accept a draw, and when you can just let go.

Managing Underperformance

As a leader you may have to manage under-performance of a trainee, a colleague or other staff. Under-performance may take several forms:

- Clinical.
- Conduct.
- Professional.

Several behaviours may warn of under-performance, especially when it comes to a trainee (Table 9.1) [35].

In dealing with under-performance [35–39], consider the following:

- View the under-performance of an individual in the wider context in which it occurs (working environment and personal life).
- Establish the true facts. Gather specifics, rather than rumours. Gather information from a wide range of relevant sources. Gather information in confidence, without ending up spreading rumours yourself.
- If there is any threat of patients' safety, then act immediately. Ensure that all measures needed to ensure patient safety are taken, and eliminate any potential harm.
- If there is evidence of criminal activity, report this to the appropriate employer's authorities and law enforcement authorities, such as the police.
- Seek help rather than acting alone. Consult the training bodies, human resources, employer.

How you approach this further and who to involve may depend on what the concerns are, and the role of the person in question (trainee or otherwise). Understand the regulations of the healthcare system in which you practise and follow these. Know the escalation pathway, if your attempts to correct things prove fruitless. However, as a start you may consider the following:

Table 9.1 Early signs of trainees in difficulty

The disappearing act: not answering bleeps; disappearing between clinic and ward; lateness; excessive amounts of sick leave
Low workrate: slowness at procedures, clerkings, dictating letters, making decisions; coming early and staying late and still not getting a reasonable workload done
Ward rage: bursts of temper when decisions questioned; shouting matches with colleagues or patients; real or imagined slights
Rigidity: poor tolerance of ambiguity; inability to compromise; difficulty prioritising; inappropriate 'whistle-blowing'
By pass syndrome: junior colleagues or nurses finding ways to avoid seeking their opinion or help
Career problems: difficulty with exams; uncertainty about career choice; disillusionment with medicine
Insight failure: rejection of constructive criticism; defensiveness; counter-challenge

From Paice [35]. Reprinted with permission

- Is there indeed a problem? Are the performance concerns something that matters, or is the behaviour within the expected spectrum and diversity one may encounter amongst staff?
- Would an informal talk help? Do not underestimate the value of an informal chat. An informal talk may elucidate what the underlying issues are and allow plans for improvement. It may also avoid unnecessary escalation of the situation which might cause a defensive behaviour and disengagement of the other party. The decision to have an informal talk may depend on whether you anticipate a successful outcome on the concerns and issues raised, and on the potential insight of the person involved. However, be prepared for those cases, where there is a real problem but no insight on behalf of the party involved. Offer the chance to an individual to explain, using open ended questions such as:

  - "How are you managing?"
  - "How are things going?"
  - "How are the on-calls? Any difficulties with the on call referrals?"
  - On occasion such simple questions may be all it takes for the walls to fall away and all issues to be revealed.

If an informal talk is unsuccessful or deemed inappropriate, then set up a formal meeting. In doing so you may consider the following:

- Inform the person as to the reason for the meeting in advance.
- Allocate sufficient time and avoid any interruptions.
- Have any relevant staff present (human resources).
- Present the facts; initially summarise and then proceed to give specifics.
- Identify underlying problem and consider plans of action:

  - Clinical knowledge or skills – close supervision, re-train
  - Behavioural attitude – close supervision, regular feedback, anger management course, communication skills course
  - Health issues – referral to occupational medicine

- Try and reach an agreement as to the need for further action.
- Set targets for improvement using the SMART model [40]:

  - **S**-pecific – what to do? whom with? where? how?
  - **M**-easurable – how many, how much?
  - **A**-ssignable – targets that can be assigned
  - **R**-ealistic – achievable given constraints
  - **T**-time related – by when? clear deadlines

Being a Follower

He who cannot be a good follower cannot be a good leader

Aristotle [1]

This chapter has up to now concentrated on managerial or leadership skills that you should aim to develop. However, the ability to be managed and follow where others lead are also important skills to acquire.

In your professional life you may end up having your own practise, or work as part of a bigger institution. Whatever the setting, it is likely that you will deal with management either directly or indirectly. Such management may be made up of other doctors, or individuals who are not medically trained, or have no clinical background. Even when management has clinical background, that background may differ from your specific clinical activities.

If you have your own practise, management could be on your payroll, but if you are an employee you may be accountable to the management running your employing institution. Even if you are "your own boss", you are still likely to be influenced by local or national healthcare policies, set out by the government or other organisations, and have dealings with the management running those. If you are in a well defined managerial or leadership post of your institution you may have to deal with those higher up, or other colleagues in the same position.

As a doctor you may concentrate on individual patient-doctor relationships, striving for high quality care. However, such relationships rarely exist in isolation. True "independent practise" is rarely encountered in many systems and countries. It is important to recognise early on that the survival of the healthcare system you are practising in, or the viability of the organisation you are employed by, may be essential, for you to be able to provide the best of care. Such survival may not only depend on doctors clinically doing their best, but also on meeting costs, meeting targets, ensuring that regulations are followed and standards are maintained, publicising the good work the institution does to make it more attractive and competitive. Many of these non-clinical tasks often have to be carried out by those in managerial positions. Hence their role and contribution should be understood and appreciated. Develop the skill of being able to see the big picture, share your institution's vision, and work along with management to improve the organisation's services.

Try and understand the management structure of your institution or other organisations you have dealings with. There may be parallel management arrangements for different employee groups, and recognising these may guide you as to whom you need to appeal to in trying to influence policies. The management structure to who the doctors report is likely to be different to those for nursing staff, theatre staff, clinic staff, or allied healthcare professionals. Hence, simply asking one of the other professionals to alter practise, may not be as straight forward as it may initially sound. Follow the management hierarchy in your requests, but also be prepared to jump up and escalate if not heard.

In dealing with management, aim for mutual respect. You may see yourself as the facilitator, who allows non clinical staff to recognise clinical priorities, but also the gatekeeper who ensures that the actions of management are always in patients' best interests.

As a follower criticise when there is a need, but also praise when things go particularly well. Question your managers or leaders, voice your concerns when they may seem to deviate from what is best for your patients, but also acknowledge and highlight their achievements and wins. Standing by your leaders when they are doing well is needed to give them the stature to fight your case, and the case of your department or organisation.

On occasion you may disagree with decisions taken or you may feel strongly that you could do things much better. But on occasion, we have to follow even when we disagree, for an institution to function, an organisation or society to stay cohesive and survive.

References

1. BrainyQuote. http://www.brainyquote.com. Accessed on 27 Sept 2014.
2. Lewin K, Lippit R, White RK. Patterns of aggressive behavior in experimentally created social climates. J Soc Psychol. 1939;10:271–301.
3. Waller DJ, Smith SR, Warnock JT. Situational theory of leadership. Am J Hosp Pharm. 1989;46(11):2335–41.
4. Waterman RH, Peters TJ, Phillips JR. Structure is not organisation. Bus Horiz. 1980;23:14–26.
5. Womack JP, Jones DT. Lean thinking. 2nd ed. New York: Free Press, Simon & Schuster, Inc; 2003.
6. Womack JP, Jones DT, Roos D. The machine that changed the world. New York: Free Press; 2007.
7. Ng D, Vail G, Thomas S, Schmidt N. Applying the lean principles of the Toyota production system to reduce wait times in the emergency department. CJEM. 2010;12(1):50–7.
8. Teichgräber UK, de Bucourt M. Applying value stream mapping techniques to eliminate non-value-added waste for the procurement of endovascular stents. Eur J Radiol. 2012;81(1):e47–52.
9. Ford AL, Williams JA, Spencer M, McCammon C, Khoury N, Sampson TR, Panagos P, Lee JM. Reducing door-to-needle times using Toyota's lean manufacturing principles and value stream analysis. Stroke. 2012;43(12):3395–8.
10. Craft RC, Leake C. The Pareto principle in organizational decision making. Manag Decis. 2002;40(8):729–33.
11. Basile F. Great management ideas can work for you. Indianap Bus J. 1996;16:53–4.
12. Juran JM. Universals in management planning and controlling. Manag Rev. 1954;43:748–61.
13. Juran JM, et al. Pareto, Lorenz, Bernoulli, Juran and others. Ind Qual Control. 1960;17:25.
14. Best M, Neuhauser D. Joseph Juran: overcoming resistance to organisational change. Qual Saf Health Care. 2006;15:380–2.
15. Kiremire AR. The application of the Pareto principle in software engineering. Ruston: Louisiana Tech University; 2011. http://tinyurl.com/Ankunda-termpaper. Accessed Apr 2013.
16. Wright A, Bates DW. Distribution of problems, medications and lab results in electronic health records: the Pareto principle at work. Appl Clin Inform. 2010;1(1):32–7.
17. NHS makes good progress on waits. BBC News. 2008. http://news.bbc.co.uk. Accessed on 26 Sept 2014.
18. Bevan G, Hood C. Have targets improved performance in the English NHS? BMJ. 2006;332(7538):419–22.
19. Gubb J. Have targets done more harm than good in the English NHS? Yes. BMJ. 2009;16:338.
20. Bevan G. Have targets done more harm than good in the English NHS? No. BMJ. 2009;16:338.
21. White C. Hunt announces drive to clear 12 month waiting list. BMJ. 2014;349:g5011.
22. OECD Stat Extracts. http://stats.oecd.org. Accessed 2 Aug 2014.
23. Results-Only Work Environment (ROWE). http://www.gorowe.com. Accessed Aug 2014.
24. Pink DH. Drive – the surprising truth about what motivates us. Edinburgh: Canongate Books; 2010.
25. Maslow AH. A theory of human motivation. Psychol Rev. 1943;50:370–96.
26. GoodReads. https://www.goodreads.com. Accessed on 26 Sept 2014.
27. Owen J. How to lead. Harlow: Pearson Education; 2011.
28. Kübler-Ross E. On death and dying. New York: Macmillan; 1969.
29. Zell D. Organizational change as a process of death, dying, and rebirth. J Appl Behav Sci. 2003;39(1):73–96.
30. The change curve. University of Exeter. https://www.exeter.ac.uk/media/universityofexeter/humanresources/documents/learningdevelopment/the_change_curve.pdf. Accessed on 26 Sept 2014.

31. Iles V, Cranfield S. Developing change management skills. London: NCCSD; 2004. https://www.ewin.nhs.uk. Accessed on 16 Aug 2014.
32. Ansoff HI. Corporate strategy. 1st ed. Harmondsworth: Penguin Books; 1965.
33. Saltman DC, O'Dea NA, Kidd MR. Conflict management: a primer for doctors in training. Postgrad Med J. 2006;82(963):9–12.
34. Kilmann RH, Thomas KW. Developing a forced-choice measure of conflict management behaviour: the MODE instrument. Educ Psychol Meas. 1977;37(2):309–25.
35. Paice E. The role of education and training. In: Cox J, King J, Hutchinson A, McAvoy P, editors. Understanding doctors' performance. Oxford: Radcliffe Publishing; 2006. p. 78–90.
36. Postgraduate medical education in Scotland: management of trainee doctors in difficulty NHS Scotland. http://www.nes.scot.nhs.uk. Accessed on 26 Sept 2014.
37. Managing trainees in difficulty practical advice for educational and clinical supervisors. NACT UK, Milton Keynes, UK; 2013.
38. The prevention, detection and management of underperformance in general practice. Department of Health, Social Services and Public Safety 2002. www.dhsspsni.gov.uk/appraisal-underperformancel.pdf. Accessed on 26 Sept 2014.
39. Mahmood T. Dealing with trainees in difficulty. Facts Views Vis Obgyn. 2012;4(1):18–23.
40. Doran GT. There's a S.M.A.R.T. way to write management's goals and objectives. Manag Rev (AMA FORUM). 1981;70(11):35–6.

Chapter 10
Obtaining the Next Post

Career progression in Medicine often involves multiple job applications for posts to help improve your clinical knowledge, diagnostic and management skills, and posts to equip you with the necessary experience for a safe practise. Even when you finish your training and you reach the final aspiring level of your career, job applications are still often essential.

Choosing, applying and successfully getting your next post, is a challenging task that requires time and effort. It requires advance planning as many posts are advertised several months in advance, and some posts such as specialisation fellowships are filled years in advance. The ability to chose and apply for the right post or training program, the ability to develop and present a clear and attractive CV and portfolio, and the ability to shine and impress in interviews, are important skills to develop. This chapter explores all these career progression areas, and gives advice how to best prepare for success. Factors that may guide you to career choice are also discussed. Finally, skills that a doctor acting as an interviewer may require, are presented.

© Springer International Publishing Switzerland 2015
C. Panayiotou Charalambous, *Career Skills for Doctors*,
DOI 10.1007/978-3-319-13479-6_10

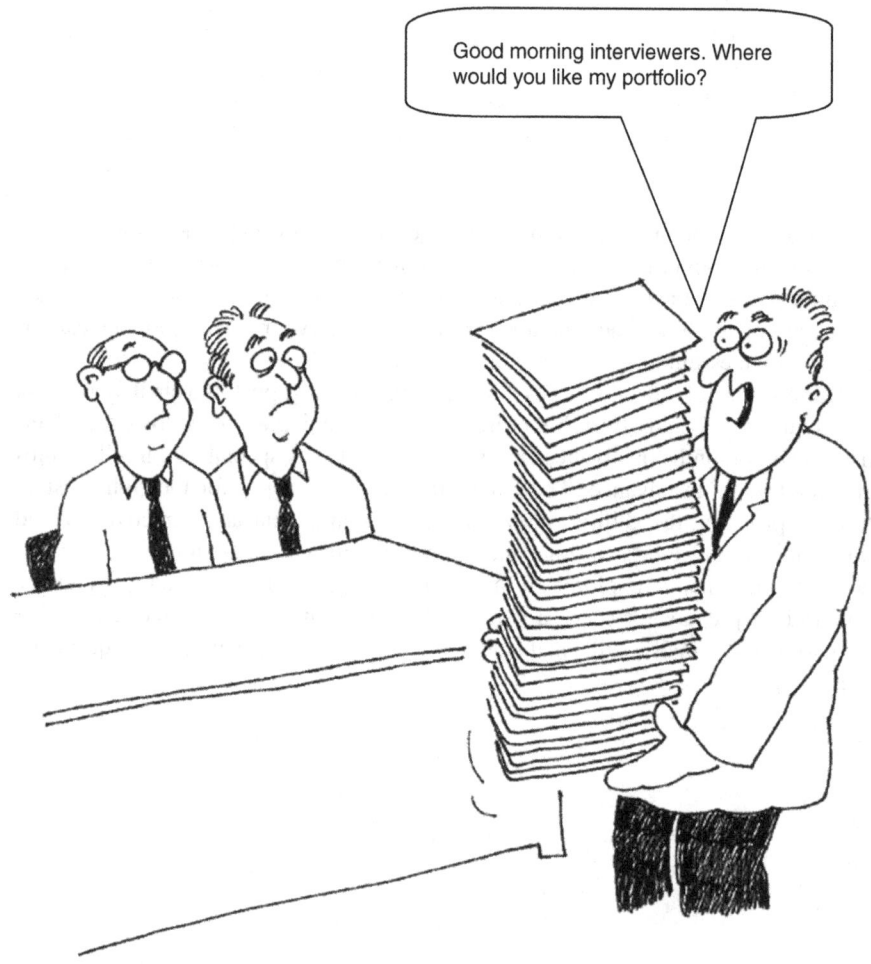

Choosing a Post

In choosing a post, first decide what you are looking for. Are you looking for a post that will help enhance your clinical training, enhance your technical or surgical skills, educate you better for upcoming exams, help you in career progression through an influential reference, enhance your research portfolio, give you better pay, or more free time. Are you looking for a post nearby, for family and social commitments, or are you able to travel and relocate where the post requires? How long are you looking to stay at such a post, and will you have to go through the re-application process after some time? These are only some of the factors to consider.

Once you decide what post you are looking for, the next step is to search for it. You may look at medical job advert sites (internet, medical journals), but valuable information about suitable posts can also be obtained by talking to colleagues and seniors. They may have done such a post in the past that are keen to recommend it, or they may be able to steer you away from non-reputable posts. They may know of suitable posts coming up before they are advertised, thus giving you the opportunity to look into them further, arrange for a site visit, and if necessary wait for them to become available.

Medical post adverts are useful for identifying a potential post, but do not rely solely on them to decide whether the post suits you. In a competitive market where doctors, particularly juniors, are highly sought after, adverts aim not only to inform potential applicants of a post, but also make the post attractive. Hence, once you identify a potential post, try and get first hand information about it. Try and determine if what the post offers is what you are really likely to get out of it:

- Will you be able to get the experience of dealing with acute medical admissions, by being the first to see such admissions when they reach the hospital, or will you be ward based and only see them once they have been dealt with and stabilised by other members of the team?
- Will you be able to attend theatre and operate, or will you spend most of time in the ward clerking elective admissions?
- Do you get dedicated time for research or are you expected to make time for it out of a busy clinical schedule?

There are several ways you may find out more about the post:

- Speak to someone who is currently doing the post, or has done that post recently. Speak to several people to get a balanced view.
- Try to visit the department and have a meeting with the person in charge of the post, to get a better picture as to how the post is viewed. If you are aware of a post coming up, arrange for such visits before the post is advertised. Once the advert goes out, visits may not be possible until completion of the shortlisting. Such a visit may increase your chances of getting shortlisted. Some candidates may simply apply to multiple relevant posts as they get advertised and only look into the details of the post only when shortlisted. Hence, it is not uncommon for some shortlisted candidates not to attend for interview. When it comes to shortlisting,

appointment panels may look not only for eligibility and qualifications, but also at how likely the person is to turn up for interview, take and start the post if that was offered. Someone who has visited the department and expressed an interest in the post, may thus have a higher chance of getting shortlisted.

Applying for a Training Program

Unlike a lone post, a training program (or rotation) is usually designed to take you through multiple posts, in one institution or multiple institutions. A local, regional or national appointment process may be utilised. Commitment to a training program may be for much longer, than that required for a lone post.

In deciding which training program to apply for you may consider:

- Will the training program provide the training you need?
- Will the training program provide the qualifications you need for progressing to the next level of your career pathway?
- Quality of training. What are the success rates of passing exams, and career progression of those completing the program?
- Specialties and sub-specialties rotated. Do they meet your specific requirements?
- Reputation of the training program.
- Is an academic pathway with both clinical and research options available?
- Requirements for successful progression. Completion and drop out rates?
- What are the requirements for entering the training program?
- How many posts are available?
- What is the usual applicant to appointments ratio?
- What is the potential competition like?
- What if unsuccessful this time, can you reapply and if yes when?
- How are the various posts of the training program allocated?
- Geographical region covered, need for frequent relocation or daily long travelling.
- Can you relocate to a different part of the country if the need arises?
- Does the training program allow career breaks or flexible working if necessary?

Applying

Once you find out as much as possible about the post and you decide that it suits you, the next step is to apply for it. Some applications simply involve the submission of your CV, whilst some may require completion of a more structured application form. You may consider the following when drawing up your CV or completing post application forms:

- Highlight your qualifications that are essential, as per the advert, for being eligible for the post. Someone reading your application should be able to identify these easily.
- Highlight your qualifications that are not essential, but are desirable for the post. Again someone going through your application should be able to pick these out easily.
- Tailor your application/CV to the specific post you are applying for. If applying for an orthopaedic post emphasise the previous posts you did in orthopaedics or other surgical specialties, rather than the time you spent as a junior doctor in respiratory medicine. If applying for a cardiology post, ensure your application gives priority to your recent cardiology audit, as compared to your audit in urology.
- Ensure that any statements on your application/CV are accurate and not overplayed or exaggerated. If anything, it is better to understate an achievement rather than endanger being accused of inaccuracies. If you are planning to do a course but have not done it yet, say so, rather than simply listing it on your CV's courses section. If the research article you submitted for publication is still under journal review, say so, rather than simply listing it as one of your publications. If you obtained a so called "green card" for performing well in your gynaecology final exams at medical school, call it so, rather than calling it a "medal" or "prize". Anything you state on your CV could be scrutinised in future interviews, and inaccuracies could raise concerns of trust and probity.
- Some application forms ask for examples where you demonstrated your ability to work as part of a wider team, ability to deal with difficult situations, ability to work under pressure, ability to lead others. Choose simple, real life examples you have experienced and which you have a lot to talk about. See the positive side of these and emphasise what you learned and gained out of such encounters. Try to avoid simply highlighting deficiencies of other players in such scenarios as they are not present to give their own account.
- Clearly state not only what you aim to gain from the post, but more importantly what you will be able to offer. You may be able to offer your ability to provide acute medical care for hip fracture patients which may thus help give better all round care in orthopaedic wards. You may be able to offer your ability to operate unsupervised and hence allow the smooth running of operating lists even when seniors are away. Alternatively, it maybe that what you offer is your ability to practise safely, your enthusiasm, and willingness to work hard and learn fast.

- Choose your referees carefully and, if possible, choose ones directly relevant to the post. If applying for an obstetrics post an obstetrician may be able to give a better account for your abilities in that field. A combination of referees that would account for both clinical and academic achievements is preferable. Better to choose referees that you have recently worked with and hence can give a more up to date account of your performance. Indeed some posts require that one of your referees must be from your last job. Consider asking any potential referees not only if they would be able to give you a reference, but also whether they would be specifically prepared to support you for the post you are applying for. Giving a reference may be different from giving a supportive reference.

CVs

One Look is Worth A Thousand Words

Fred R. Barnard [1]

CV Format

The exact format and layout of your CV is a personal preference but the following may be considered:

- Keep it simple and succinct, easy to read.
- Avoid long text paragraphs.
- Clear and easy to read font.
- Consistent use of font type and size.
- Avoid excessive use of bolds, italics, underlining, colours.
- Consistent use of subheadings.
- Present events (jobs, publications) in reverse chronological order (most recent first). Particularly, when it comes to jobs, make it very clear as to what your current post is, followed by previous posts.
- If possible start each section on a new page or middle of page, rather than at the last page line.
- You may modify the sequence of presenting information, particularly research, audit, teaching, or management, according to the type of post or role you are applying for. For example if applying for a research post, give your previous research experience priority, putting it after your medical posts. If applying for a management position, give your previous managerial experience priority, putting that after your medical posts.

CV Content

The content of your CV will depend on what you have done up to that point and what level of your postgraduate career you are at, but the following may be included:

- Personal details: name, contact details.
- Qualifications – professional exams, postgraduate, undergraduate.
- Academic achievements – prizes, honours, distinctions, awards.
- Hospital posts –

  - Current post
  - Previous posts

You may include a summary of your job duties for each post, such as on-call commitments.

- Postgraduate education – courses, meetings, conferences.
- Membership of professional bodies –

  - National medical organisation, medical indemnity organisation, postgraduate colleges, specialty societies

- Research –

  - Publications – give full reference
  - Submitted articles under review, articles in preparation, ongoing research

For each project give the names of the collaborators, with your name and their names in the order they would appear in any future publication.
- Audit –

  - Initial audit, re-audit, closed the loop audits
  - May give a brief summary of standards assessed, results, and change in practise

- Teaching and other educational activities –

  - Whom you taught
  - Format of delivering teaching (one to one, small group, lecture, course)
  - Regular or opportunistic

- Administrative/managing experience

  - Management courses attended
  - Management duties – such as on call rota master, organising journal club

- Other positions of responsibility –

  - In work
  - Out of work

- Interests – anything unique, anything to stand out?
- Referees –

  - Names
  - Position
  - Contact details

Portfolio

Portfolio is a collection of evidence of academic or career progression [2–4]. Unlike your CV which summarises your achievements, the portfolio contains evidence to support each of those. The portfolio should be thorough yet succinct. You may consider the following sections as a generic order, along with examples of supportive documents for each:

- Personal details.
- Contents page.
- Qualifications – original university or exam certificates.
- Academic achievements – certificates of prizes.
- Hospital posts – certificate of completion of pre-registration years, training program.
- Postgraduate education.

  - Personal development plan – statement
  - Certificates of courses or meetings attended
  - Appraisal meetings – confirming documentation
  - Assessments of competence – completed work based assessments
  - Logbook of procedures

- Membership of professional bodies – up to date certificates of membership.
- Research – copies of full articles published (or at least the first page of those), copies of abstracts published. For presentations given in meetings a copy of the program showing details of the presentation, and a copy of the slides of the presentation fitted on a single page.
- Audit – if presented, a copy of the slides fitted in one page, or a letter from the audit lead confirming the audit was done.
- Teaching and other educational activities –letter from head of teaching confirming those activities, copy of slides, feedback from students.
- Administrative/managing experience – confirming letters from head of department or other seniors, short description of role, achievements of that role.
- Other positions of responsibility – confirming letters from relevant authorities.
- Interests – supporting certificates such as violin grade reached, martial arts belt obtained.
- Feedback from colleagues – structured feedback or letters.
- Feedback from patients – survey result, complaints (summary of complaints received, action taken and outcomes), compliments – copies of thank you letters, cards.

If going for an interview, ask whether there is a marking scheme for portfolio which gives marks according to various domains, and adjust the filing of your portfolio as per those domains. It should be easy for an interviewer to extract information from your portfolio for marking purposes, rather than having to go back and forth through the folder.

It may be that portfolio marks are given for demonstrating your team building skills. This may involve examples from multiple areas such as running a research team, carrying out a multi-centre audit, organising a vene-puncture course for medical students, running the resuscitation team. Rather than expecting the assessor to search for these in the research, audit, teaching and management domains, make a new domain labelled as "team skills" containing confirmation of all the above activities.

Shortlisted for Interview

Give me six hours to chop down a tree, and I will spend the first four sharpening the axe
Abraham Lincoln [5]

- If shortlisted for an interview, consider asking again for a visit to the department and, if possible, a meeting with members of the interview panel. Whether this is allowed or forbidden may vary from institution to institution. However, there is no harm in enquiring. Such a visit could allow you to have any remaining questions clarified. It may also give you and interviewers alike, the opportunity of meeting outside the artificial and often stressful environment of an interview. Such visits may further help to show that you are truly keen and enthusiastic about the post, as you have taken the effort and time to explore the working environment and its people. If applying to posts far away from your current base, or applying for a post abroad, the above may be achieved over the phone or over the internet.
- Apart from visiting members of the medical team consider also meeting members of the extended team, such as nursing staff, management staff, rota-master, all of whom may be able to give you an all round picture of the post.
- Have a look around the hospital or practise where the post is located to see how would you feel working in that environment? Is it a brand new modern hospital with nice surroundings, where you can enjoy nice lunch at its lustrous restaurant, or is the roof leaking and are the walls peeling? Does the place lift your spirit or does it make you feel miserable? Is it near the countryside with its long weekend hikes or near the city centre with its buzzing nightlife?
- If the post involves relocating explore any potential accommodation that you may have to take. Will it be liveable by your standards, and will it be affordable? Is accommodation provided along with the post? Does the post assist with relocation expenses?

The Interview

Eighty percent of success is showing up

Woody Allen [5]

Performing well at an interview relies on adequate communication skills, knowledge, but also, importantly, thorough preparation. Interviews can be in various formats, including panel interviews or station interviews. In panel interviews, a candidate is interviewed by a panel of interviewers who may take turns to ask questions. In station interviews, a candidate attends multiple stations, each of which concentrates on a particular area. The latter is similar to OSCE stations that you may have encountered in your undergraduate exams. In panel interviews, the whole panel sees and can thus assess the whole of your interview performance, whereas in station interviews, the interviewers of each station are usually not aware, at that stage, of your performance in other stations.

Interview questioning may take several formats. You may be asked questions that look for direct succinct answers, or look for more elaborate, logically structured thinking and answering. You may be asked to interpret medical charts, investigation results, or demonstrate your technical and surgical skills. There may be role playing, whereby you are asked to take a medical history, break bad news, counsel or consent. You may even be asked to solve a non-medical puzzle! Keep a broad mind and expect the unexpected!

Know your CV and application inside out but take a hard copy with you, to refer to if necessary. Take with you a hard copy of your portfolio and any documentation that would support the accuracy of your CV and application form.

Make sure you know where the interview is taking place, and give sufficient time to be punctual. It is easy to get lost in massive hospitals, where all corridors look alike. Even if you work at the institution where the interview is carried out, treat the interview itself as if taking place away from your usual workplace. Taking some time off from a busy clinic, or attending the interview after a night on call, may not work out as planned.

Before you enter the room ensure that your mobile phone is silenced. Introduce yourself and shake hands if offered. Stand next to the chair and sit down when asked to do so. Try and keep calm, smile, look and sound pleasant, appear determined. Speak slowly, confidently, be concise. Answer in a polite way, using formal but simple terms. Maintain an upright posture and eye contact with the panel members. Avoid distractions, avoid looking through the window. If interviewed by a panel, answer looking at the person asking the question, but intermittently look and address the other panel members too.

If you have not understood the question, ask if the interviewer could re-phrase it. If asked about a topic, a recent political event or policy, that you are have no knowledge of, say that you are not familiar with it and ask for some more information. The examiner may be able to give you more information to allow you to answer the question. Often, what is looked for is an opinion or a logical approach to a problem, rather than knowledge per se. Avoid making up terms or words that may not even exist.

You may be asked about controversial issues. You may be asked about the role of staff not medically trained as theatre assistants, about shortening the length of training, or other controversial issues. Be open minded even if you have strong personal views. Look at both sides of an argument, both positives and negatives. Try and give the positive side, then address the downside, and finish on a positive note. This may indicate ability to compromise, and a positive attitude even to difficult situations, important attributes for the workplace.

Look and behave professionally. In particular, dress for the occasion and keep formalities. It maybe you know some of the panel members, they may be working with you, they may know all about your work, but they still ask about it. Answer such questions as if each panel member has not met you previously, assume they do not know anything.

Areas that may be examined in a medical interview include:

- Portfolio – what stage of your career are you at, previous undergraduate and postgraduate education, what previous posts have you done, how much clinical/surgical experience do you have, what technical/surgical skills have you acquired, what can you do with minimal supervision, have you kept a logbook for technical/surgical skills, logbook of assessments of clinical skills?
- Achievements – what achievements are you proud of, honours, merits, distinctions, prizes, exams. Say what you are proud of and why.
- Commitment – examples that demonstrate your commitment to the specialty, such as went into hospital in free time, joined the doctor on call, or attended extra operating lists in free time to improve surgical skills.
- Research – what research have you done, which is your best research project and why, what have you published, what presentations have you given, what is the value of research, should clinicians get involved in research? In choosing which of your research studies to describe as your best, consider using the one highest up on the research ladder; it may be more difficult for interviewers to argue against a randomised trial rather than a large case series, even if you spent more time and effort in the latter.
- Audit – what is audit, what is the difference between audit and research, what audits have you done, which was your best audit and why, did you initiate or lead the audit, did you do the initial audit, re-audit and close the loop, how did you improve practise? If you have closed the loop in one audit, then better talk about that.
- Clinical scenarios – scenarios that may be encountered when on duty, emergency scenarios. What would you do, when would you inform your seniors? Start from the basics, ALS, or ATLS guidelines [6, 7] rather than jumping to the obvious problem. Show that you have a system in your approach, keep an open mind, demonstrate you are safe, that you will not miss something important.
- Management – examples demonstrating your managerial skills, examples of closely working with management.
- Why you? Why should you get the post? What will you bring to the post?
- How much homework have you done about the post, what do you know about the post? What do you know about the department? Why are you applying for this post?

- Alternative plans – What plans do you have if you do not get this post? Are you applying for other posts? Alternative plans, do not necessarily mean that you are looking around and you are not committed to the post you are applying for. Instead, they may show you recognise that there is always a chance of not getting the post, no matter how good you are, and you have a contingency plan if that were to happen. Make it clear that you are not someone who will give up, simply because you were unsuccessful in your particular post application, but someone who is determined to pursue their goals, and will live to fight the next day.
- Questions – it is not unusual for the interview to end by being asked if you have any questions to make. Have a question prepared. However, if your queries have already been answered by all those you met and spoke to previously, it is acceptable to say so. This may not be the best time to ask whether you could be paid through your offshore company in Monte Carlo.

Try and anticipate questions. Write down potential questions, and prepare answers to them. Practise answering these questions Ask a friend or your partner, to ask you questions and answer them as if in a real interview. Ask for their feedback. Construct answers that are short and simple. Try and answer, as when you speak to your peers or seniors on a day to day basis, rather than using complex language. Avoid using unusual terms or language that you do not normally use, and hence will be difficult to remember and recall.

No matter how the interview went, thank the panel, stand, shake hands, if offered, and walk out closing the door behind you.

You may be told of the outcome at the end of the interview or you may be contacted at a later stage. Try and find about that from the administrative staff prior to the interview. If offered the post, be clear as to whether you want to accept it or not. If you applied for other posts and you want to wait for their results, say so, and ask for time to consider before giving your final answer. It is not considered appropriate to accept the offer, simply to turn it down shortly afterwards. If you do that, you may still be required to start your post and work your notice time.

Even if you do not get the post, it maybe useful to ask for feedback. It maybe that you were up to scratch, but a better candidate happened to turn up. Alternatively, it maybe that there are weak areas on your CV that could be improved, or interview skills that could be further polished.

In interviews, like exams, there are things that we can control and things that we can not. You can improve your qualifications, you can build up your portfolio and boost your CV, you can anticipate and practise answering potential questions. However, there will be the odd question that you have not thought of, something unexpected. Accept this and aim to reduce the unexpected to as minimum as possible.

Starting a New Post

The very first step towards success in any occupation is to become interested in it
William Osler [5]

You were successful and got the post of your choice. Any new post, any change, is a challenge, but certain actions may help smoothen that transition. Before you start you may consider:

- Visit your future senior or department to remind them of your arrival. This may be the time to mention upcoming leave, inform them that you may be in induction for a couple of days at the start, or that you are starting on nights, so they do not keep looking for you, wondering where you are.
- Speak to the person currently doing your future post. What are the exact duties, what is the normal week like? What should you be particularly careful about? Any tips as to what the seniors like? What do they dislike?

When turning up for the post there may be a formal induction, a structured way of introducing you to the institution, the department and the post. However, even if a formal induction does not take place some information is important to establish early on:

Consider asking:

- Who can you ask for help? Do you refer medically unwell patients to the outreach intensive care unit team, the acute medical team, the anaesthetist? Whom do you refer to during normal working hours? What about during on calls?
- What is the distinction between specialties? What gets referred to acute medicine, cardiology, geriatric service? What gets referred to plastics, orthopaedics, general surgery?
- Why if an emergency arises? Where do we keep the crash trolley, the pelvic external fixator, the compartment pressure monitor, the cardiac pacing equipment?
- What procedures can be done in the Emergency Department and what must be referred on?
- What ages do we take? Do we admit young ones or do we send them to the specialist children's hospital?

Shortlisting and Interviewing

> I've learned that people will forget what you said, people will forget what you did, but people will never forget how you made them feel
>
> Maya Angelou [8]

As a doctor you may attend interviews, not only as an interviewee, but as an interviewer too. You may interview applicants for a junior post, a colleague, employee, or even a more senior post. The task may feel daunting. What questions to ask? How to be fair? How to choose the best? Give your role the seriousness it deserves. Someone's career, progression or well being may be at stake. As with all other tasks you may undertake, follow the rules, treat all as equal, be consistent, open, and transparent.

Consider the following if shortlisting or interviewing for a post:

Shortlisting

- Define essential and desirable qualifications.
- Establish a clear marking scheme.
- Keep good documentation of the reasoning for shortlisting or not shortlisting an applicant.

Interviewing

- Practise how you will be asking questions – wording, tone, sequence.
- Avoid behaviours that disrupt candidate (answering phone, chatting to other panel members).
- Body language – should you be leaning backwards, hands behind head, when asking questions, should you be shaking head, pulling hair in response to every wrong answer?
- Keep good documentation of applicants responses.
- Clear marking scheme. What would you consider the pass mark to be? What should an excellent candidate get?
- Transparent marking scheme.
- Similar questions may help differentiate candidates.
- Avoid body language or expressions that may make the candidate uneasy. Do not humiliate or make fun of the candidate.
- Disclose relations with candidates follow the rules as what to do if you know one of the candidates.
- What if candidate has no response? How do you move on?
- What if they give a wrong answer? Do you correct the candidate or say nothing and just move on?
- What if you know a candidate? Do you excuse yourself and ask someone else to interview or continue as normal?

Choosing Specialisation

Don't feel guilty if you don't know what you want to do with your life. The most interesting
people I know didn't know at 22 what they wanted to do with their lives. Some of the most
interesting 40-year-olds I know still don't

Mary Schmich [9]

Becoming a doctor is only the first step in your long term career. Soon after
graduation you may need to make a decision as to which career path to follow. You
may want to become a generalist, a specialist, or even a subspecialist. You may want
to look after little people, young persons, elderly people. You may like short encounters with patients, or may thrive at establishing long close relations. You may want
to become a physician, a surgeon, a pathologist. You may want to be hospital based,
community based, lead a huge team, or be a one person team. You may want to
leave clinical work altogether, decide to become an academic, work for a commercial company, a pharmaceutical company, a medical indemnity organisation.

Apart from the above, in deciding which career path to follow you may also
consider:

- Will I enjoy that job?
- What is the job likely to be? Is it a stressful or easy going environment?
- What are on call commitments like?
- I am I good at this? Play to your strengths. If you enjoy talking to patients is
  pathology the best career? If you do not like technical skills should surgery be
  your first choice?
- Intensity of work.
- Working hours.
- Remuneration.
- Training required, length, intensity, need to pass postgraduate exams, need to
  take time out for postgraduate research, or postgraduate degree. How competi-
  tive is it to get into a training program?
- Career path, career breaks.
- Chances for employment. How competitive is it likely to be? However this may
  not be the a very reliable indicator as the job market may change, and where
  there is shortage today there may be a surplus by the time you complete your
  training.
- What if I decide to practise in a different part of the world?

To help you decide you may:

- Speak to various people doing the specialty, at various stages of their career to
  get a balanced view. Speak also to those not in the specialty, to get an outsider's
  view.
- Work in the specialty you want to follow, in as high a grade as possible, before
  committing to it. The picture we may get of some specialties as medical students
  may be distorted. Not all specialties get a fair balance in medical school, and
  often we do not really know what working in such specialties involves. Similarly,

the picture you may get as a very junior doctor, who is mainly ward based may not be truly representative of the overall job. Do on calls, in that specialty, see how busy they are.

- If you can not work in the specialty you are considering, shadow someone who does, to get a real taste of what it involves.
- Work with different teams and people before you finally decide. You may have a good time in one attachment because your seniors are easy going and very supportive. However, you may have a completely different experience if working with a not so supportive team. The opposite is also true, as a bad experience does not necessarily mean that is the specialty or career area to blame.

You may still be undecided, not sure what to do. Others around you may have a clear plan, others may really know where they want to be, and what they are working to. Take time, do not rush. You are likely to spend more years in the final career you chose as compared to your training, hence make a good decision. Consider taking some time working in a generic post such as the Emergency Department, or the intensive care, where you may acquire transferable skills that can be of use in many of the possible career pathways you are considering.

References

1. The phrase finder. http://www.phrases.org.uk. Accessed 26 Sept 2014.
2. Jenkins L, Mash B, Derese A. Development of a portfolio of learning for postgraduate family medicine training in South Africa: a Delphi study. BMC Fam Pract. 2012;13:11.
3. Tochel C, Haig A, Hesketh A, Cadzow A, Beggs K, Colthart I, Peacock H. The effectiveness of portfolios for post-graduate assessment and education: BEME Guide No 12. Med Teach. 2009;31(4):299–318.
4. Saltman DC, Tavabie A, Kidd MR. The use of reflective and reasoned portfolios by doctors. J Eval Clin Pract. 2012;18(1):182–5.
5. BrainyQuote. http://www.brainyquote.com. Accessed 26 Sept 2014.
6. Resuscitation Council (UK). Advanced life support. 6th ed. London: Resuscitation Council (UK); 2011.
7. American College of Surgeons; Committee on Trauma. ATLS: advanced trauma life support for doctors (student course manual). 8th ed. Chicago: American College of Surgeons; 2008. ISBN 10: 1880696312.
8. Goodreads. http://www.goodreads.com. Accessed 26 Sept 2014.
9. Schmich M. Chicago Tribune, 1997. http://www.chicagotribune.com. Accessed 26 Sept 2014.

Chapter 11
When Things Go Wrong

No matter how hard we work, how well trained and committed we are mistakes do happen, and on occasions things do go wrong. Often it is not an individual but the underlying system to blame, the underlying processes or lack of them.

The ability to respond appropriately when things go wrong and the ability to investigate and address such events, to minimise the chance of them occurring again, are important skills to develop. An approach for dealing with adverse events is initially presented. The root cause analysis methodology is then introduced with the five Whys and cause-effect methods discussed. The skills of learning from mistakes, encouraging a no blame structure, and recognising error prone situations, are explored. Ways of dealing with complaints, malpractise or medicolegal action, are also presented.

© Springer International Publishing Switzerland 2015
C. Panayiotou Charalambous, *Career Skills for Doctors*,
DOI 10.1007/978-3-319-13479-6_11

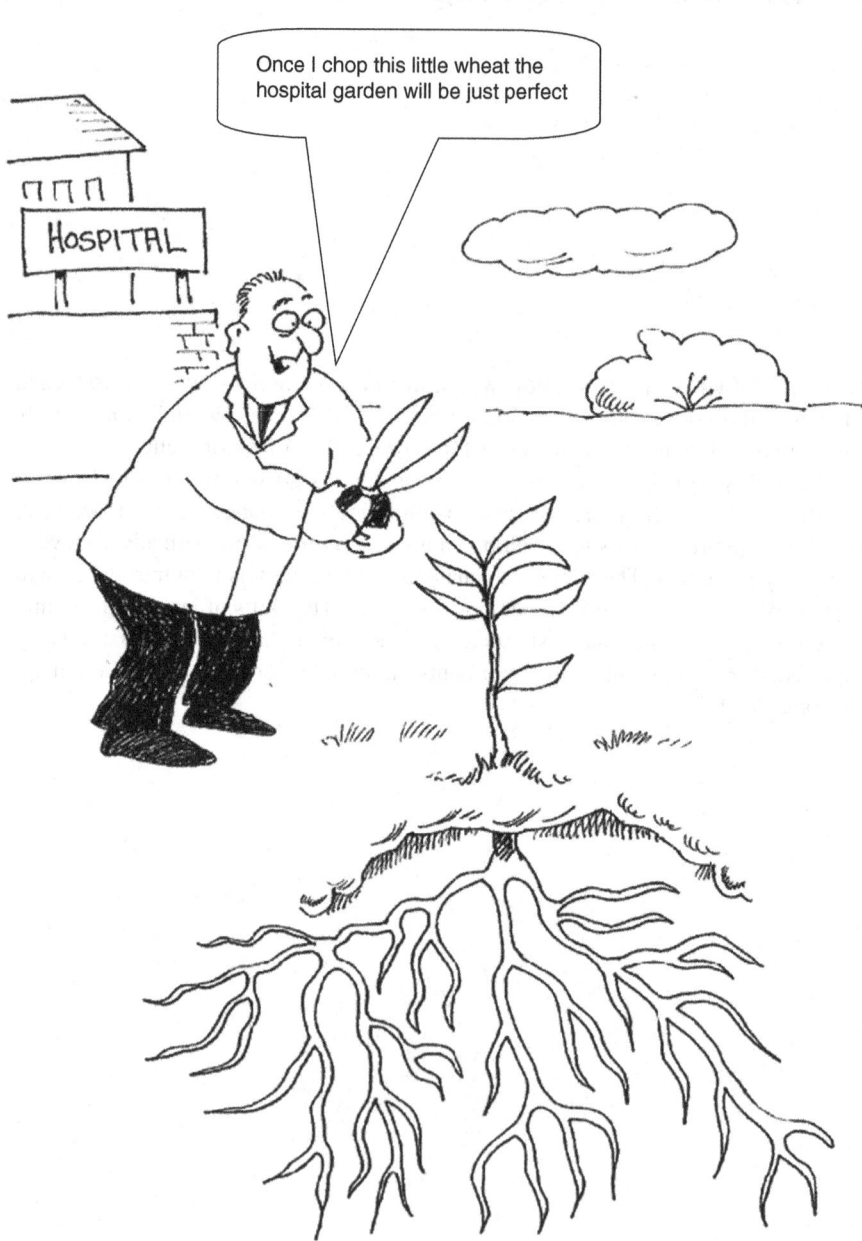

Managing Adverse Events

As a clinician you may encounter or be involved in a medical error or adverse event. The World Health Organisation defines adverse events as "an injury related to medical management, in contrast to complications of disease. Medical management includes all aspects of care, including diagnosis and treatment, failure to diagnose or treat, and the systems and equipment used to deliver care" [1].

Administration of the wrong medication, transfusion of incompatible blood or blood products, pressure ulcers due to inadequate hydration and skin care, wrong site surgery, infection due to failure of antibiotic prophylaxis, clostridium colitis due to unnecessary prolonged antibiotic treatment, failure to pick an early tumour on a mammogram, not recognising malignancy on a skin biopsy, are only some of potential adverse events that may be encountered in clinical practise.

About 10 % of patients in acute hospitals in the developed world may experience one or more adverse events, with about 50 % of these being potentially preventable (Table 11.1) [2–5]. A study evaluating hospital patients in Portugal, reported that 10.8 % died and 5.4 % experienced permanent disability as a result of an adverse event. In the USA the total national costs due to adverse events are estimated at 4–6 % of national health spending [6].

Being able to deal with an adverse event is an important skill to develop. You may have to deal with such an event in the acute setting, when this is first recognised, or you may contribute to investigating the event and determining what went wrong and the reasons behind it.

An approach used by the author and described using the acronym SAFEST (Stop, Antidote, Find, Explain, Sorry, Transform), may help you deal acutely with a harmful event. This is summarised below:

Table 11.1 Incidence of adverse events in hospitals in developed countries, and proportion of these considered to be preventable

Country	Incidence (%)	Preventable (%)
UK [2]	10.8	52
New Zealand [3]	11.3	61.6
Portugal [4]	11.1	53.2
Denmark [5]	9	40.4

S-top any further harm from occurring, discontinue the inappropriate medication, inappropriate fluid administration or blood transfusion.

A-ntidote any harm that already took place. Reverse any damage that has been done. Treat the venous thrombosis that occurred due to failure to prescribe thrombo-prophylaxis, reverse with fresh frozen plasma the anticoagulation effect of inappropriate anticoagulant administration, reverse the opioid overdose.

F-ind why this happened. Root cause analysis. Why did the error happen? What is the underlying cause? What system failures allowed this to happen?

E-xplain the event to the patient or relatives as needed. Be open and transparent.

S-orry. Sympathise to the patient for what went wrong and apologise if there is any specific regret, oversight or mistake.

T-ranform your practise to ensure the harmful event is un-likely to happen again. Learn from the event and introduce long lasting prevention changes. Make plans as how to deal with such an event if it were to reoccur.

Find the Real Cause

To make no mistakes is not in the power of man; but from their errors and mistakes the wise
and good learn wisdom for the future

Plutarch [7]

In analysing what went wrong try and get to the bottom of things. If you do not
identify the real underlying cause, then you will only be addressing its manifesta-
tions. As in Medicine, you will be treating the symptom rather the underlying disor-
der. Root cause analysis is a term used to describe this approach. It does not
concentrate on the most apparent cause of an adverse event, but explores what lies
beneath. It has been used extensively in the engineering and aviation industry and
more recently in healthcare.

Multiple investigation systems have been described to help examine adverse
events. The five Whys (Fig. 11.1) [8] and the cause-effect analysis (Fig. 11.2) [9]
are two of these. These try to put structure into the investigation of the underlying
problems. Both suggest that, when things go wrong, it is often not due to an individual's fault, but due to absent or poorly performing underlying processes or
systems.

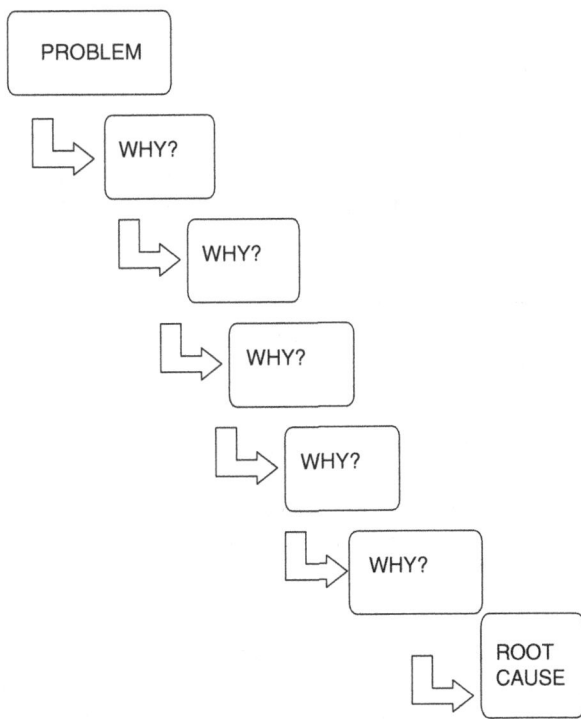

Fig. 11.1 The five whys
approach for root analysis
(Based on Taiichi [8])

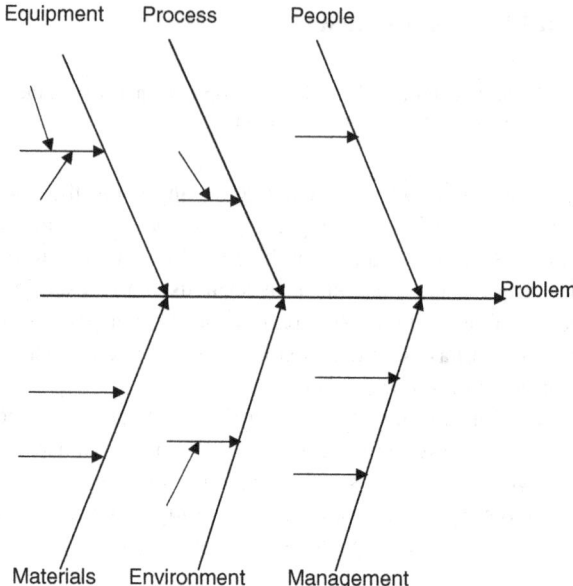

Fig. 11.2 Fishbone diagram used in root analysis of an error or adverse event (Based on Ishikawa [9])

The Five Whys

The five Whys was initially described by Taiichi Ohno, pioneer of the Toyota Production System, to help identify problems in the manufacturer's production line [8]. In this method, you keep asking "why?", until you get to the root of the problem, and identify the process that needs rectifying, to ensure similar events are not repeated. The answer to one "why?" usually leads to a further "why?" until the bottom cause is reached. The number 5 is only arbitrary and a smaller or larger number of "why?"s may be needed to get to the real cause, depending on the problem examined.

An example of the five Whys approach may be:

- Patients are waiting too long in the emergency room – Why?
- Junior doctors take too long to see them – Why?
- Not enough juniors doctors roistered – Why?
- New doctors not recruited on time – Why?
- Advertisement for new doctors delayed – Why?
- Advert posted rather than emailed to advertising journal.

The root problem in this situation was that traditional posting was used for setting up an advert for junior doctors. An upcoming post-office strike was not taken into account. Unless prompt advertising and appointment of juniors occurs in the future, the same problem is likely to reoccur.

Cause: Effect Analysis

The cause and effect diagram (also known as Fishbone diagram due to its shape or Ishikawa diagram as credit to its initial descriptor) provides a structured way of assessing the underlying causes of a problem.

This was originally described by Professor Ishikawa at the University of Tokyo [9]. It looks at the problem, and classifies its potential causes into groups of factors, that may account for the problem occurring. Such factors may be:

- Available resources (materials).
- Surrounding environment and context.
- Management and supervision.
- Equipment.
- Processes, pathways and protocols.
- People involved.

The cause and effect diagram is presented as a horizontal line pointing to the problem (the hard backbone of the fish!) with branches or sub-branches (lesser bones!) arising from this, and pointing to potential causes. Just dealing with the obvious hard backbone is not enough. One must find and remove the small, but sharp tiny bones, to avoid further choking trouble!!

The initial step is to write down the problem, and then brainstorm, to gather information as to the possible real causes. The five Whys method can be used alongside Ishikawa's cause-effect diagram to get to the bottom of each contributing factor.

Learning from Mistakes

From the errors of others, a wise man corrects his own

Publilius Syrus [7]

Developing the skill of encouraging a no blame structure and learning from mistakes, may help avoid further similar adverse events or errors. Being able to recognise error prone situations, and hence approach these appropriately, may also minimise the risk of adverse events.

Encouraging a No-Blame Culture

Accept that mistakes will happen, things will go wrong, even in healthcare. James Reason, Professor of psychology at the University of Manchester, UK, and author of the book, "Human Error" [10], stresses the importance of acknowledging the role of both individual and systemic failures due to an error or accident occurrence.

James Reason suggests that, normally, there are several layers, or barriers, that protect against an error. Each of these barriers may have potential holes or weaknesses. If one barrier fails, the next barrier may provide protection. However, if the weaknesses of several barriers coincide, then an error may occur. This is known as the Swiss cheese model (Fig. 11.3), whereby each barrier acts like a slice of Swiss cheese, each slice having one or more holes (inherent weaknesses). Catastrophic

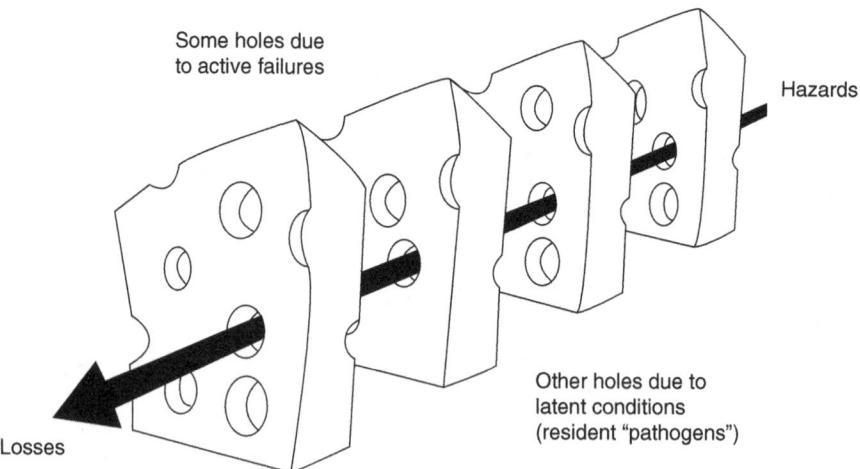

Successive layers of defences, barriers and safeguards

Fig. 11.3 The Swiss cheese model or error causation (From Reason et al. [11]. Reprinted with permission)

failure may occur, when the holes of multiple adjacent slices align, and thus nothing can stop the error passing through [11, 12].

When an error occurs, the tendency is to immediately blame frontline staff or an individual, blame their specific actions (active failures). However, it is important to recognise that usually there are underlying weaknesses in the system (latent conditions) that must be identified and addressed [13–15]. Hence in root analysis, one must look at both the actions of individuals but also the effectiveness of the underlying barriers, the underlying systems, processes, pathways.

Use adverse events as stimulators for addressing system defects, rather than opportunities for blaming individuals. Reason challenges as myths the concepts that bad things (errors) happen only to bad people, that people freely choose to behave and act in unsafe ways, and that errors occur randomly. Reason stresses that errors can happen even to the best individuals, that choosing between safe and unsafe behaviours is not simply a matter of an individual's free choice but is often influenced by the context in which events occur, and that errors often follow certain, anticipatable patterns.

Reporting of adverse events, or near misses, can help us learn from each other's experiences and has reduced errors in the aviation industry. In the preface to the World Health Organisation's draft guidelines on adverse event reporting, Sir Liam Donaldson, Chair of the World Alliance for Patient Safety, raises the orange wire-test as a way for promoting safety in healthcare [1] and questions:

> Imagine a jet aircraft which contains an orange coloured wire essential for its safe functioning. An airline engineer in one part of the world doing a pre-flight inspection spots that the wire is frayed in a way that suggests a critical fault rather than routine wear and tear. What would happen next? I think we know the answer. It is likely that – probably within days – most similar jet engines in the world would be inspected and the orange wire, if faulty, would be renewed. When will health-care pass the orange-wire test?

The recent problems encountered with Boeing's Dreamliners' lithium batteries and the grounding of the planes shortly after launch, until technical issues were resolved [16], help remind how accurate Sir Donaldson's words are.

Learning from the experiences and encounters of other individuals, departments or organisations is invaluable. We all learn from our mistakes, but we may not afford to learn solely from our own mistakes.

A no-blame culture where the individual does not feel threatened, may encourage disclosure of adverse events, errors and near misses, and help encourage dissemination of such experiences. Heard et al. [17] surveyed anaesthetist consultants and residents in Victoria, Australia. Amongst 433 respondents, the statement "doctors who make errors are blamed by their colleagues" was the one that most respondents considered vital in discouraging the reporting of adverse events due to error. Fear of litigation, blame, fear of getting into trouble, disciplinary action, not wanting the case discussed in meetings and unsupportive colleagues, were also perceived as barriers to reporting adverse events. Having senior colleagues who openly encouraged reporting was considered one of the most favoured factors promoting disclosure of adverse events.

Fig. 11.4 The three bucket model for recognition of error prone situations (Based on Reason [18])

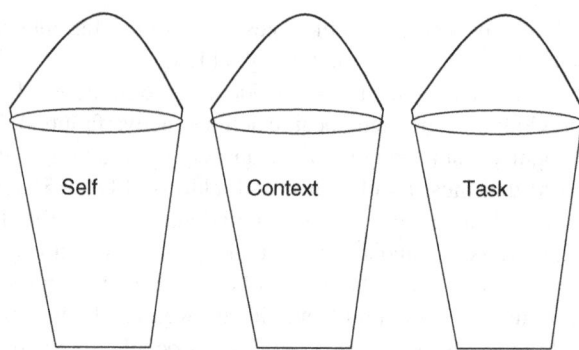

Aim for a no blame culture, where individuals are encouraged to come out and report what went wrong, viewing this as a learning lesson rather than trying to hide their mistakes. Learning from mistakes and putting systems in place to minimise the chances of mistakes recurring should be the main priority.

James Reason stresses the importance of:

- Accepting that errors can occur and will occur.
- Assessing potential hazards before commencing a task.
- Have plans to deal with any encountered problems.
- Seek help as needed.
- Checking the experience and knowledge of colleagues or other staff, especially if they are strangers to you.
- Avoid false assumptions.

Develop the ability to recognise situations with a high probability of error occurrence. Reason proposed the three bucket model [18] (Fig. 11.4) for recognising, and hence appropriately approaching situations, that have a high potential for error occurrence. One bucket relates to the current state of the participant (limited knowledge, inexperience, being sick or tired), the second to the context in which the task occurs (lack of time, interruptions, malfunctioning equipment), and the third to the error potential of the task per se (complex task, multiple steps). Bad stuff in each bucket should make alarm bells ring, concentrate attention and focus minds.

Complaints

...God created the world in six days. On the seventh day, he rested. On the eighth day, he started getting complaints. And it hasn't stopped since

James Scott Bell [19]

At some point in your career it is likely that a patient, relatives, other staff or someone else may complain about you. Indeed complaints in healthcare seem to be on the rise [20–22]. It may be a complaint about attitude, inadequate communication, clinical judgement, clinical management, unnecessary waits, cancellation of treatment, the list is endless. Complaints may arise, no matter how professional, clever, careful, or committed you are. Complaints may be verbal or written, informal or formal. Patients may complain asking for explanations as to what happened or an apology for what occurred. The complaint may aim at enforcing accountability or ensuring that bad experiences are not faced by others.

Receiving a complaint against you can be a difficult and stressful event. As doctors we may work hard, strive for perfection, aim to give the best we can. Yet a complaint may cause anxiety or self-doubt as there may be an implication that you did not give your best. A complaint may cause fears of personal consequences, damage of reputation, impact on time and resources.

Try and shine a bright light on a dark situation. View a complaint as feedback, as an educational learning exercise, as a positive rather than a negative event. It may be time consuming investigating and responding, but it is an opportunity to identify potential weaknesses or deficiencies in your practise. It may be an opportunity to further improve yourself and practice. Can you learn from it? Can the complaint help you gain knowledge, experience, or wisdom?

In guiding you as how to handle a complaint, try and remember, what you expected, last time you complained about a matter outside work – about that parcel that went astray, your car which broke down shortly after its annual service, the hotel room which did not meet what the advert said, the bank overcharge, the restaurant food that was not fresh, your passport application which has still to come through. In dealing with such complaints you might have expected to be listened, understood, taken seriously, be given a prompt response, a clear explanation and action that would rectify the situation. If these are the standards we may set for non health matters, should we not at least aim for similar standards when it comes to resolving complaints of healthcare issues?

You may consider the following in dealing with a complaint:

- Do not belittle the complaint, no matter how insignificant it may sound, no matter how obvious the explanation may be. It is important enough to the person complaining.
- Deal with it in a professional way. Organisations are often judged by the public in the way they deal with complaints. How can one be persuaded that an organisation or individual are doing their best, when even a complaint process is not handled to the highest standards?

- Give a prompt response. Acknowledge the complaint promptly and reply that you will investigate and give a response. If you fail to acknowledge it or give a delayed response you may give the impression, rightly or wrongly, that you are avoiding it. If you seem to be running away from the complaint someone could infer that you have something to hide. Set a target time for giving a response to the complaint and stick to it.
- Break down the complaint into specific questions that can be more easily dealt with.
- Investigate by obtaining reports of those who were involved.
- Reply to the complaint using plain language that a non medical person can easily understand.
- Resolve rather than escalating a tense situation. You may not be able to reach an agreement, your account of events may be different to the complainant's account, your messages may not be getting through, you may have different opinions as to how things should be done, and your explanations may not suffice. Do not be antagonistic, do not pick a fight. You may simply acknowledge that you disagree.
- Seek help from your seniors or other appropriate authorities of your institution (such as complaints department) to guide you in how to deal with a complaint.
- Seek emotional help from friends and colleagues if you are finding the experience too hard.

The five Es approach (Establish, Empathise, Explain, Embark, and Escalate) used by the author, may help you put a structure as to how to handle a complaint. It may help you deal with a verbal complaint in clinic or the ward, construct a written response to a formal complaint, or plan and run a complaint resolving meeting.

E-stablish: establish the exact complaint. What is the complaint about? Establish the facts. Why is the complaint happening? What went wrong? Take into account all available information and listen to the complainant's story. Their account may differ from yours. Identify the events for which you and claimant agree.

E-mpathise: express your sorrow for what happened. Express your understanding of the complainant's concerns, of what they are going through.

E-xplain: give your explanation as to what happened and apologise for what went wrong or for what could have been done better, if applicable. Make it clear where things went right but try and explain why these were not perceived so. Explain any learning points for yourself or the organisation, and changes put in place to ensure things are not repeated.

E-mbark: on the future with a clear agreed plan with the complainant, if such a plan can be reached. This may involve an agreed acceptance that the issue has been resolved, an agreed plan for further management, or agreement that there is still disagreement.

E-scalate: inform the patient as how the complain can be taken further if still no resolution. What other avenues are available at local or higher level, how can they be accessed?

Legal Action

Fall seven times and stand up eight

Japanese proverb [7]

And if you thought that dealing with a complaint is challenging enough, what if you find yourself in the middle of legal action for medical malpractice or negligence. The chances of being in the centre of a medical malpractice action are high, being higher in some specialties and some parts of the world than others. Jena et al. [23], in the New England Journal of Medicine, looked at malpractice claims against physicians of different medical specialties in the USA and estimated a cumulative risk for being sued at least once for malpractice by a given age. Overall, each year of the study, 7.4 % of doctors had a claim and 1.6 % had a claim leading to an indemnity payment. There was variation of the risk amongst specialties, being highest in neurosurgery (19.1 %) and lowest in psychiatry (2.6 %). Thirty-six percent of physicians in low risk specialties, and 88 % of those in high risk specialties, were projected to have their first claim by the age of 45. Seventy-five percent of physicians in low risk specialties, and 99 % of those in high risk specialties were projected to have a claim by the age of 65 (Fig. 11.5).

You may be informed of a malpractise action either directly or through the legal department of the organisation or institution you are practising in. Being in the centre of such action can be a difficult and stressful event. Like complaints, malpractise actions may carry a huge burden in terms of time, and fears of damage to one's reputation. Malpractise actions may also lead to defensive Medicine.

It is important to acknowledge that legislation risks exist, no matter how careful and safe we are. Anticipating these may equip you better to deal with them when they arise:

- Maintain good documentation which you can refer to if needed.
- Practise safe but do not let the fear of ligitation guide your management.
- Seek advice from the legal department of your institution or defence union at the earliest opportunity.
- You may be asked to give your version of events. Give a factual report referring to the documentation in the patient's notes.

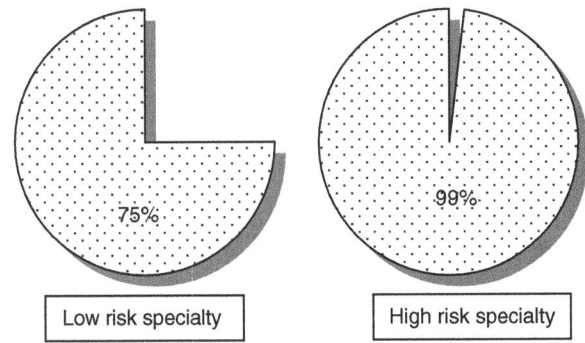

Fig. 11.5 Estimated proportion of physicians facing a claim by the age of 65, according to specialty risk (Based on Jena et al. [23])

- If you recall events which happened, but were not documented at the time, write a report of these and keep it for your own records, as you may refer to it if needed at a later stage. Under no circumstances modify or change the patient's records, as it may be viewed as an attempt to falsify those.
- Speak to family, friends and colleagues about your worries of a legal action, without disclosing details of a particular case. Emotional support and a listening ear maybe of great help in such situations.

You may want a quick resolution but in some countries, and some legal systems, such actions may take a long time to resolve, especially if the claim is to be contested. Seabury et al. [24] analyzed data from 40,916 physicians covered by an insurer in the USA, and found that the average physician spends 50.7 months (equivalent to about 11 % of an assumed 40-year career) with an unresolved, ongoing malpractice claim.

References

1. Leapec A. WHO draft guidelines for adverse event reporting and learning systems. From information to action. Geneva, Switzerland: World Health Organization; 2005.
2. Vincent C, Neale G, Woloshynowych M. Adverse events in British hospitals: preliminary retrospective record review. BMJ. 2001;322:517–9.
3. Davis P, Lay-Yee R, Briant R, Ali W, Scott A, Schug S. Adverse events in New Zealand public hospitals I: occurrence and impact. N Z Med J. 2002;115:203–9.
4. Sousa P, Uva AS, Serranheira F, Nunes C, Leite ES. Estimating the incidence of adverse events in Portuguese hospitals: a contribution to improving quality and patient safety. BMC Health Serv Res. 2014;14(1):311.
5. Schioler T, Lipczak H, Pedersen BL. Incidence of adverse events in hospitals: a retrospective study of medical records: Danish study of adverse events. Scan J Public Health. 2000; 32:324–33.
6. Institute of Medicine (IOM). To err is human: building a safer health system. Washington, DC: National Academy Press; 2000.
7. Brainyquote. http://www.brainyquote.com. Accessed 26 Sept 2014.
8. Taiichi O. Toyota production system: beyond large-scale production (English translation ed.). Portland: Productivity Press; 1988.
9. Ishikawa K. Guide to quality control. Tokyo: Asian Productivity Organization; 1976.
10. Reason J. Human error. Cambridge, UK: Cambridge University Press; 1990.
11. Reason JT, Carthey J, de Leval MR. Diagnosing "vulnerable system syndrome": an essential prerequisite to effective risk management. Qual Health Care. 2001;10 Suppl 2:ii21–5.
12. Reason J. Human error: models and management. BMJ. 2000;320(7237):768–70.
13. Reason J. Safety in the operating theatre – Part 2: human error and organisational failure. Qual Saf Health Care. 2005;14(1):56–60.
14. Reason J. Human error: models and management. West J Med. 2000;172(6):393–6.
15. Reason J. Understanding adverse events: human factors. Qual Health Care. 1995;4(2):80–9.
16. Dreamliner. Boeing 787 planes grounded on safety fears. BBC news. http://www.bbc.co.uk/news/business. Accessed on 26 Sept 2014.
17. Heard GC, Sanderson PM, Thomas RD. Barriers to adverse event and error reporting in anesthesia. Anesth Analg. 2012;114(3):604–14.
18. Reason J. Beyond the organisational accident: the need for "error wisdom" on the frontline. Qual Saf Health Care. 2004;13 Suppl 2:ii28–33.
19. Goodreads. http://www.goodreads.com. Accessed 26 Sept 2014.
20. Iacobucci G. Complaints against the NHS in England reached 3000 a week last year. BMJ. 2013;30:347.
21. Triggle N. Written complaints about care in the NHS rise by 8 per cent. Nurs Manag (Harrow). 2012;19(6):6–7.
22. Mead J. Trends in surgical litigation claims. Ann R Coll Surg Engl. 2014;96:180–3.
23. Jena AB, Seabury S, Lakdawalla D, Chandra A. Malpractice risk according to physician specialty. N Engl J Med. 2011;365(7):629–36.
24. Seabury SA, Chandra A, Lakdawalla DN, Jena AB. On average, physicians spend nearly 11 percent of their 40-year careers with an open, unresolved malpractice claim. Health Aff (Millwood). 2013;32(1):111–9.

Chapter 12
Looking After Yourself

As a doctor, as a dedicated professional, it may be easy to get absorbed into hard work and ignore yourself, your health, your social life. Work patterns with shift duties, in hospitals with limited food options, long working hours, sleep deprivation, work pressures and stressful situations, can be detrimental to your work-life balance.

The ability to devote time to relax, eat well, exercise, and keep a healthy, balanced lifestyle, are important skills to develop. This chapter addresses these issues and stresses the importance of looking after yourself. At the same time it discusses how to approach controversial situations as well as the need to join a workforce union and a medical protection body.

The sketches (figures) included in this article were drawn by Robert Brownlow, commissioned by CP Charalambous. The copyright is held by CP Charalambous.
Copyright of Acronyms SAFEST, LOAD, 5Es, are reserved by CP Charalambous.

© Springer International Publishing Switzerland 2015
C. Panayiotou Charalambous, *Career Skills for Doctors*,
DOI 10.1007/978-3-319-13479-6_12

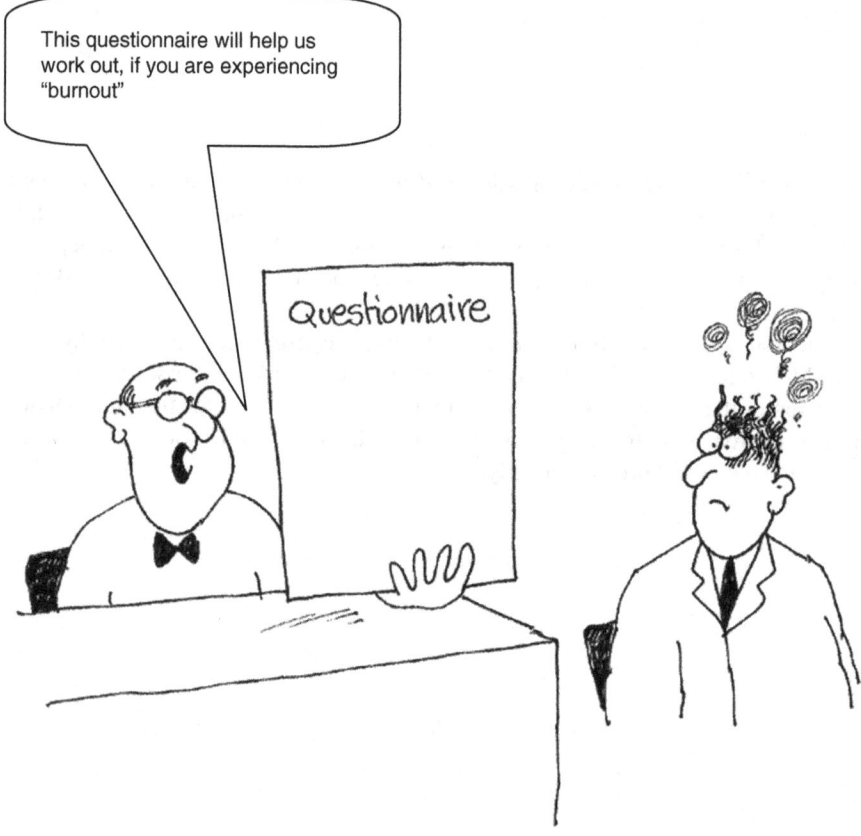

Personal and Private Time

The time you enjoy wasting is not wasted time

Bertrand Russell [1]

- Does sharing your social life with all at work help bonding with colleagues or do you prefer keeping your personal life private?
- Do you thrive at the challenge of sorting out work matters anytime of the day and night or do you want your out of work time to be truly yours?
- Does receiving work emails in your private account allow you to stay on top of work or do such emails stop you from relaxing when off duty?
- Does receiving a phone text from your senior about a bright research idea make you feel a valued team member or would you rather not be disturbed whilst out on a romancing date?

Whichever route you choose will be right as long as this is what really full fills you and gives you mental and physical peace. Work life balance is truly a balance but make sure you set the balance. It is your work and it is your life. Like anyone else you are entitled to your personal time, your private life, you worked hard, you earned it.

If you decide that private life is private and personal time is personal, then stick to your ground and demand that. Others may want to know all you get up to when not at work, as it is a good talking point for their lunchtime gossip. Others may feel you should be available to their requests at any time; you may be well paid after all. But you make the decision as how much you can give.

The car manufacturer Volkswagen agreed to stop sending emails to some of its employees when they are off-shift, following complaints of disruption of family life and burnout. Other companies, such as Henkel the maker of Persil washing powder, announced an email "amnesty" between Christmas and New Year, with messages sent to its workers only in emergencies [2, 3]. According to recent French rules, during out of office hours employees in the digital and consultancy sectors will have to turn off their work phones and avoid opening work email, and firms cannot pressurise employees to check messages [4].

Work life balance is what it says. Asking for respect of your personal time is not a sign of lack of motivation or lack of enthusiasm. In contrast, it may signify that you are an all round human being who has interests and an enjoyable life outside work.

Eating

Too many people just eat to consume calories. Try dining for a change

John Walters [1]

As a doctor you may a lead a busy schedule, often having to eat on the go. You may work unsocial hours or shift patterns when most food outlets are closed. You may practise in hospitals or other health care institutions, away from city centres and food stores, with limited food purchase options. There is often much publicity about the quality and nutritional value of hospital food available to patients, yet little is said about what food is available for staff and visitors. Take aways, food vending machines, hospital cafeterias, and restaurants, with processed food that is rich in sugars, fat, and calories may soon become a way of life.

The Hospital Nutrition Environment Scan for Cafeterias Vending Machines and Gift Shops is a scoring system assessing hospital food providers. It takes into account factors such as the availability of healthy foods, prices of healthy as compared to un-healthy foods, and promotion of healthy foods [5]. A recent study utilising this scoring system examined 39 hospitals in Southern California, USA, and found that hospitals scored poorly, achieving on average only one quarter of the maximum possible score points. Only 15 % of cafeterias surveyed kept unhealthy foods away from the checkouts [6]. A survey of hospital cafeterias' managers in New York, USA, showed that less than one third of respondents had training in nutrition, and less than one quarter of hospital cafeterias followed nutrition standards for their food [7]. Simon Stevens, the chief executive of National Health System (NHS) England recently stated that "A lot of the food in hospital canteens, not just for patients, but for staff is chips and burgers" and promised plans of healthier food in NHS hospitals [8].

Eating well and having a balanced diet, is part of healthy life. Look after yourself, and make healthy choices when it comes to food. It may mean preparing and taking your own food from home or taking time to walk out of hospital to a place for a healthy lunch. Invest the time and put in the effort needed.

Sleeping

There is a time for many words, and there is also a time for sleep

Homer [1]

Medical care is a 24 h calling. At some stage of your career you may work at night as part of shift work or on-call duty. Night work, shift work and prolonged hours can disrupt your circadian rhythm, cause sleep deprivation and fatigue. Our body's circadian rhythm runs over a period of about 24 h and is influenced by changes in light and dark. Working at night or trying to go to sleep during the day means fighting against this circadian rhythm. Most of us need about 8 h of sleep a night and if any lost sleep is not repaid soon afterwards, fatigue may ensue [9].

Sleep deprivation and fatigue may lead to poor performance, impair professionalism, undermine safety, and reduce learning. Sleep deprivation may lead to depression and hurt life quality. Shift work is associated with an increased risk of cardiovascular disease; elevation of blood pressure, dysrythmias, and increased blood cholesterol during and after night shift are well documented [10–25].

But even classical 24 h on call duties can lead to an increased risk of cardiovascular disorders. Baldwin and Daugherty looked at sleep deprivation and fatigue during residency training. They reported that residents getting fewer than 5 h of sleep per night, were more likely to report serious accidents or injuries, conflict with other professionals, and significant medical errors. They also had an increased chance of being named in a malpractise suit [26].

A working group of the Royal College of Physicians of London, published simplified, well written advice, as to how to prepare for, survive and recover from a night shift [9]. Their advice can be summarised as follows:

Preparing for a night shift

- Establish a good sleep routine. Get extra sleep before the first night shift (go to sleep early the night before, lie in late the morning prior to shift).
- Have a 2 h afternoon nap before the first shift.

During a night shift

- If possible, take 20–45 min naps rather than simple relaxation breaks. Avoid sleeping for longer durations to maintain alertness upon awaking.
- Eat regularly (prior to coming on duty, halfway through and at end of shift).
- Get exposed to bright light during nightshifts, such as light lamps.
- Avoid excessive caffeine.

Recovering from a night shift

- Consider the risks of driving after a night shift. If you have been up all night do you really need to hit the motorway or should you get some sleep first? The increased risk of motor accidents amongst interns and residents following a night shift is well reported.
- Get to sleep as soon as you get home.

- Sleep well during the day.
- Pay back your sleep debt as soon as feasible.

If you are about to start a stretch of night shifts, plan as how to tackle it. Do not underestimate the effects of shift work, long duties, lack of sleep. Catch up on your days off, lead a healthy lifestyle, look after yourself.

Exercise

Take care of your body. It's the only place you have to live

Jim Rohn [1]

Exercise regularly, keep healthy and fit. As doctors we well know the benefits of exercise, both physiological and psychological. We advocate such benefits when it comes to advising patients, yet we may not ourselves do as we preach.

In the UK, the department of health recommends that an adult does 30 min of exercise at least five times a week [27, 28]. Shorter bouts of exercise may have an accumulative benefit, similar to single bouts. However, Gupta and Fan [29] evaluated the exercise patterns of junior doctors in England and reported that only 21 % met these exercise recommendations. This proportion was much lower than the national average of the general population of a similar age group which was at 44 %. Interestingly, 64 % of this cohort of doctors met the guidelines as medical students. Lack of time was cited as the most common cause of not participating in regular exercise, followed by lack of motivation and lack of facilities. Similar findings have been reported in other parts of the world. A study of resident physicians in the USA, found that the likelihood of being overweight increased with the year of training [30]. A survey of medical consultants in Ireland, found that one in five took no exercise [31]. Only half of Catalan physicians surveyed exercised regularly, and 57 % of male physicians reported being overweight or obese [32]. A survey of primary health care professionals in Saudi Arabia, reported only 40 % having a normal body mass index, and only 21 % being physically active [33].

A doctor's job is often a sedentary job, even in those specialties that you might consider very active. Josephson et al. used pedometers to assess the number of steps taken by Emergency Medicine residents, in the USA [34]. They tried to determine if these residents satisfy the daily walking recommendations of the Centres for Disease Control and Prevention [35–37]. They reported that 90 % of residents did not meet the target number of steps for their shifts. This may come as a surprise to someone who has watched "ER" [38].

It may be easy, in a busy medical schedule, to overlook regular exercise and keeping fit. Over exhaustion and fatigue, due to a hectic workload, may also be important contributing factors. Participation of residents and fellows at the Mayo clinic in Rochester, Minnesota, in a team based, incentivised exercise program, was shown to significantly improve physical activity and life quality [39]. A trend towards reduced burnout was also observed. Consider the following in ensuring that you keep active and fit:

- Allocate time for exercise, the gym, for a run, for playing tennis or golf, or for any other physical activity you really fancy.
- Join the hospital gym or exercise classes if available.
- Take the stairs rather than the lift.
- A brisk walk down the hospital corridor may help if nothing else is possible.

Supportive Friends

Lots of people want to ride with you in the limo, but what you want is someone who will take the bus with you when the limo breaks down

Oprah Winfrey [1]

Have good supportive friends. Friends will be there in difficult times when pressures are mounting. Friends will be present when you need them, put in the time and effort, it is a worthy investment. It is easy in a busy doctor's schedule, with unsocial working hours, to lose contact, to drift apart. You may work when others are out partying, you may be revising when others are relaxing. Make an effort to keep in touch, to keep connecting lines open.

It is not uncommon to mainly have friends from work, meet and talk about work, discuss those challenging cases you dealt with, boast about those clinical signs you picked, those rare diagnoses you made, moan about the management pressures and other job hassles. Having friends at work helps interpersonal relationships, lets you see the human side of each other, and provides an understanding ear for what you daily go through.

However, having friends outside work, of different professions, interests and backgrounds, is of great value too. It may help you keep in touch with the rest of the world, keep in touch with reality. You may be complaining that your study leave budget is reduced, when your high school mate has no job to go to. You may be boasting about your new surgical skills, when your best friend is proud of her new Tango skills. You may be worried about not getting a place in the surgical skills course, when your friends are worried about not getting tickets for the next derby match.

Have lots of friends, keep old ones and make new. Have an interesting life.

Look After Your Health

A sound mind in a healthy body Satire X of the Roman poet

Juvenal [1]

How can you give the best to your patients if your own health is failing? As doctors we may be reluctant to seek medical advice for our own health, we may self diagnose, try self prescribed remedies, hope that with time all will get better. We may seek corridor consultations from peers and colleagues rather than following the formal routes. There may be several reasons for this; not wanting to disrupt our routine or take time off work, fearful of making it known to others, concerned about the risk to our career.

Amongst doctors registered in Barcelona, 49 % reported not having a family doctor. Fifty-two percent had asked colleagues for health advice, but only 48 % followed their suggestions and 82 % admitted self-prescribing [40]. Amongst 4,198 medical practitioners registered in Hong Kong who responded to a postal questionnaire, two-thirds looked after themselves when they were last ill, with 62 % self-prescribing medications [41]. Amongst New South Wales doctors in Australia only 42 % had a general practitioner, and most self-prescribed. Of these 18 % reported emotional disorders, 3 % alcohol problems and 1 % drug abuse. However, not many discussed such problems with their doctor. Although 26 % had a condition that needed a medical consultation, they felt inhibited from consulting a doctor [42]. In the UK 10–20 % of doctors may become depressed during their career. Rates of addiction to drugs, alcohol abuse, and suicide are also alarmingly high [43, 44]. In a survey of about 8,000 surgeons in USA, 30–50 % reported burnout, anxiety or depression. Six percent had experienced suicidal thoughts, with those having made a medical error, being more likely to have such thoughts [45].

McKevitt et al. surveyed general practitioners and hospital doctors in the UK [46]. Amongst more than 1,200 respondents, about 85 % reported having continued working when it might have been better to take sick leave. Factors cited as reasons for working through illness included having work that could not be delegated, fear of burden to colleagues, commitment to the job, disapproval of taking sick leave, and costs for covering absence. Perkin et al. assessed whether junior doctors in a teaching hospital in the UK stayed at work inappropriately, whilst having an infectious illness (such as gastrointestinal disturbance, upper respiratory tract or skin infection) [47]. More than 60 % of junior doctors continued to stay at work during such an illness episode. Concern about colleagues having to do more work, perceived pressure from seniors, and the belief that the illness would not influence their ability to work and would not be transmitted, were cited as reasons for such behaviours.

If you are not well should you be going into work? Is it worse to take time off, or find your self in a situation where your performance is suboptimal and can not offer the best to your patients? If you were picking a flight what would you think if the pilot turned up with bad flu, sneezing, coughing, shivering? Would you feel proud of the pilot for putting duty above self, or would you be really worried about your safety and question the judgement?

As a doctor you may be dealing with patients' safety, or directly with patients' lives. You may be reluctant to take time off, being concerned about your patients whose appointments may have to be postponed, your peers who may have to cover your on call, your seniors who may have to cope without you, the potential financial loss. But if you are not well should you be really going to work?

Dealing with Stress

There's going to be stress in life, but it's your choice whether to let it affect you or not
Valerie Bertinelli [1]

Stress may be considered a reaction to outside demand and pressures. A certain level of stress is good for maintaining alertness. Indeed, as the stress efficiency curve suggests, low levels of stress may lead to higher productivity. However, as stress levels rise and pressure mounts, performance and productivity may drop, leading to the typical inverse U curve (Fig. 12.1) [48–50].

Being a doctor often carries high pressures. The high workload, need for speedy decisions, implications of actions taken, dealing with life and death, breaking bad news, challenges of career progression, awkward or competitive colleagues, continuous professional development, constant evaluations and exams, are only some of the potential stressors. Stress can build up and have adverse effects, leading to negative feelings, loss of enthusiasm and motivation, memory difficulties, lack of concentration, mood swings, and sleep loss.

Lam et al. [51] assessed the psychological well being of interns in Hong Kong and found that about one third experienced abnormal levels of depression, anxiety and stress. Long working hours, being frequently called during a night shift, and high workload, were cited as the most important stressors. Holidays, peer support and sleep, were quoted as giving substantial stress relief.

Prolonged high level of stress can lead to a pathological state known as burnout. Occupational burnout has three components, which may coexist at various levels of severity [52]. These are:

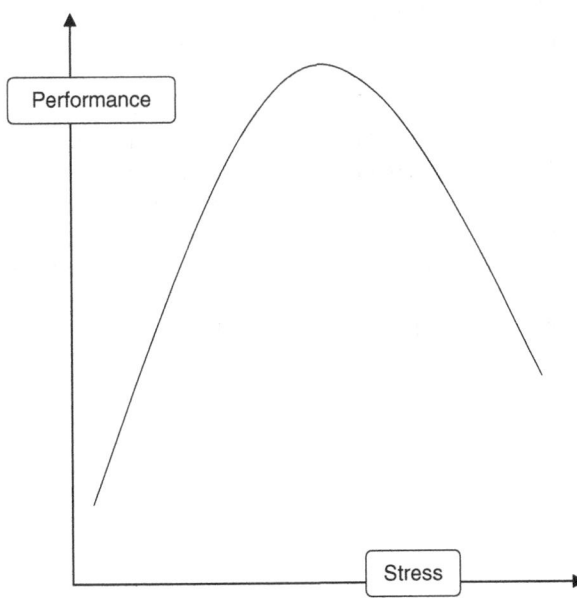

Fig. 12.1 The stress performance curve (Adapted from Diamond et al. [50])

1. Emotional exclusion, whereby an individual's energy levels are depleted.
2. Depersonalisation, whereby an individual gets detached from the job, with feelings of cynicism predominating.
3. Feelings of inefficiency, feelings of lack of personal achievement.

Christina Maslach, Professor of Psychology at the University of California, developed a structured measure of burnout, known as the Maslach burnout inventory [53]. This has been used to assess burnout rates in different professionals. Using this inventory, about 30–70 % of physicians, oncologists, surgeons and obstetricians, have been reported to experience burnout [54–60].

Trying to analyse the aetiology of burnout, Leiter and Maslach [61], developed a model which described the degree of match or mismatch between an individual and six domains of their working environment. They considered that the greater the mismatch, the greater the risk of burnout. Understanding the domains where mismatch occurs can help target potential interventions. These domains are:

- Workload – excessive workload.
- Control – lack of control of one's working environment.
- Reward – reward of work not matching expectations.
- Community – poor relations with colleagues and other staff.
- Fairness – lack of perceived fairness with regards personal development, promotion.
- Values – values of the organisation may not meet or may contradict individual's core values.

Deal with stress, do not crumble under it.

- Identify the stressor. Is it a person, behaviours, events, volume?
- Can you eliminate the stressor?
- Can you change your response to the stressor? Think of the bigger picture. Is this worthy getting so worried, so concerned about? A look at the "pale blue dot", a photo of Earth, taken by the spacecraft Voyager from 3.7 billion miles away on its journey to the unknown [62], may help you put all in perspective.
- Find healthy coping mechanisms to help you relax. Do something you really enjoy to get your mind away from all pressures. It may be you enjoy swimming, running, watching a movie, going to the opera, going to the pub, going out clubbing. Try and switch off, devote time to your self, away from thoughts of work.
- A well balanced diet, social support, comforting relationships may truly help.
- Avoid unhealthy coping mechanisms (alcohol, caffeine, smoking).

Ask for Support

You are never strong enough that you don't need help

Cesar Chavez [1]

We may all go through difficult times in life, and doctors are not immune to these. It may be your father is unwell and your really worried about his health, it may be you just had a new baby which keeps you up all night, it may be you are between houses sleeping on the floor until the new mattress gets delivered, it may be your parents are splitting after 30 years together, or your own partner is leaving you for someone else. If you have personal troubles that affect your work performance, consider being proactive and asking for help.

A young resident in a famous institution was once contemplating not to attend his grandfather's funeral, as he was worried that taking time from work might be frowned upon by seniors. A friendly chat with a secretary made him realise that not attending his grandfather's funeral might be something to always regret. It made him realise that his seniors would, if anything, be very supportive of him. Asking for help is not a sign of weakness, but a sign of an individual being a strong professional, being able to recognise and acknowledge that a problem exists. Is it better to admit such problems when others question your performance, or disclose them yourself first? Unless you divulge such problems, others will not know. You may view your seniors as high flyers, ambitious, strict and demanding players, but after all they are all human beings, whose years of life experiences should allow them to offer the necessary support. Speak to your colleagues, peers, seniors, employer. Discuss the problem, ask for advice and help. Look with them for solutions, coping mechanisms.

It may be that you need to take some time off, it may be that your work intensity needs to be temporarily reduced or it may be that you need to be given a substantial work task to help take your mind away from worries. Different situations and different individuals may require custom made solutions. Acknowledging the problem, letting others know, is the first step towards a solution.

Do Not Bite Off More than You Can Chew

It is kindness to immediately refuse what you intend to deny

Publilius Syrus [1]

Sometimes you may be overwhelmed with work and yet more tasks may be thrown at you. Consider the following situations:

- You are in a full time clinical post, whilst revising for the upcoming membership exams, finalising the thesis for your Masters, organising the journal club, planning the juniors' weekly duty rota, and preparing for your upcoming appraisal. You have just finished a week of night shifts, you are tired, short of sleep, feel exhausted and you are asked to cover the next weekend on call as overtime, double the normal pay.
- You are leading a randomised research trial at your current hospital whilst you are writing up an article for publication, and getting ready to present in your specialty's annual scientific meting. You just started a new post, you are finding your feet in the wards, and your new boss asks you to lead a new exciting multi-centre study.
- You are leading a busy clinical service, your week is filled with clinical commitments, and the hospital director asks you to take on the management of the whole department.

If it is too much do not take it on. If you are going to lose your sleep over it, politely decline. Learn to say no. If you find the volume, or level of work is affecting your well being, then reconsider. Should you be cutting down, should you be refusing any additional tasks? In a diplomatic way you can explain why you are unable at the moment to take anything else on. If you could take new tasks on, only by dropping other activities then say so. If you could take new tasks on, only if additional resources became available then ask for those.

If you refuse, the person you are refusing to may be momentarily disappointed, but, if wise, will understand that is the reasonable course of action. Is it better to be honest and refuse or take it on and not deliver?

Stay Away from Controversies

Integrity has no need of rules

Albert Camus [1]

As a doctor you may encounter situations where decisions are controversial, where right and wrong may not be immediately apparent. Consider the following situations:

- A knee replacement course is run in the skiing resort of Davos. You will be attending, and your employing hospital will pay for your return flight to Davos, as part of your study leave budget. You are considering taking a week annual leave at the end of the course to spend it skiing there.
- A pharmaceutical company is offering to fly you to the sunny island of Santorini for an international meeting, where the early results of its new anti-hypertensive drug will be presented. Seafront accommodation for you and your partner is included. You are considering whether to accept the offer.
- You will be attending a medical meeting in London and accommodation is paid by your employing hospital. The hospital's accommodation office is booking your stay, and offers you two hotels to choose from. Both are close to the course venue, one is a 4 star hotel at £200 a night, and the other a chain brand hotel at £70 a night. You are contemplating as to which one to choose.

The ethical, legal and philosophical arguments, as to what is the right approach, in the above and other similar controversial situations could be endless [63]. Follow the rules of your institution, the rules of your overseeing medical body, follow the law of the land.

However it is also worth considering whether just following the rules is sufficient. Is it just the letter or also the spirit of law that matters? What would your patients think if they knew? What would the general public think? What would you think had you been an outsider, rather than the central player? If such practises were questioned, are you prepared to go through the process of having to justify your actions, or would such a defence process cause you distress and upset? The decision as to what to do is yours.

Medical Indemnity

In the end, you have to protect yourself at all times

Floyd Mayweather [1]

No matter how knowledgeable, careful, and committed we are, things may still go wrong. Patients may not only complain, but also take legal action asking for compensation. Legal action may also be taken even when things have not gone wrong, but such claims still have to be defended. Legal action may cause unbearable stress, and legal expenses can impose a huge financial burden, potentially leading a doctor to financial ruin. Seabury et al. [64] analyzed defence costs, associated with 26,853 malpractice claims, made between 1995 and 2005 among 40,916 physicians in the USA. They reported that the average (±standard deviation) cost associated with such claims was \$22,959 (±41,687). Claims in which an indemnity payment was made had higher defence costs than those resulting in no payment (\$45,070 vs. \$17,130). Hence these authors demonstrated that there is a substantial cost of defending even those cases that never result in a payment.

Medical indemnity aims to provide cover for such legal actions. It is essentially a form of insurance, to help cover legal defence and representation costs and also make compensation payments. Consider the following situations, where medical indemnity cover may become essential:

- If you work for the government or a hospital your employer may provide indemnity for the work you do for them. However, the legal department of such employers aims to protect your individual needs but also the organisation's needs, and the two may not always coincide. Additional help may come in handy.
- You may do additional work to that of your regular employer's or may be fully self employed.
- Someone may collapse on your holiday flight or in the street. As a good Samaritan you may rush to their help, only to find yourself in the receiving end of legal action.
- You may be attending an inquest for a patient's death, a potentially daunting experience, even for the most hard-hearted. Advice and support may help you meet the challenge.
- Someone may have complained to the press about your performance, and your face is flashed all over the news. You may need a spokesperson to put forwards an alternative view.
- You may be giving a written response to a complaint, and need independent advice on its structure and wording.
- You may be facing ethical or legal dilemmas at work, and need additional advice and help.
- You may be facing disciplinary action taken by your employer, or overseeing medical body, for your clinical or non-clinical conduct, and need advice, support or representation.

Which medical indemnity provider you choose may depend on what is available, which part of the world you practise, the stage of your career, and what you exactly need from cover. Factors to consider in making such choices are:

- Amount covered. Is there limit or an excess?
- Length of cover, if you were to leave the provider.
- Length of time that legal action can be taken against you after an event.
- Indemnity arrangements required by your regulating medical body.
- Will you be covered definitely or is cover discretionary?
- Is any other support provided? Are training about legal aspects of Medicine, assistance with the press, assistance with disciplinary hearings provided?
- Does it cover all aspects of your work? Such as treating high demand patients like sports professionals, or high risk patients?
- Does it cover only clinical work, or does it also cover report writing, such as medico-legal reports?

Medical indemnity helps protect you in difficult times, but equally important, it ensures that your patients will not be disadvantaged and left short of compensation if harm were to happen. Appreciating the value of medical indemnity and choosing the one that meets your needs, is a skill to develop.

Chaperoning

Depending on your speciality and your exact medical role, you may have to perform intimate examinations of patients such as pelvic, or breast examinations. Some examinations may not be so intimate but may require partly undressing a patient, such as listening to a patient's chest, examining a patient's hip, palpating the abdomen for tenderness, examining the spine. You may have to palpate a patient's hands for tenderness, or feel the groin, knees or feet for pulses. You may test leg sensation, as part of neurological examination.

A third party, a chaperon, present in such examinations, helps to protect the patient and provide reassurance that nothing untoward happens. Medical regulatory bodies, specialist societies, and medical indemnity organisations, advise for the use of chaperones in intimate examinations, but previous studies showed that their use is often sparse [65–67].

Rosenthal et al. [65] reported that only 37 % of surveyed general practitioners in the UK had a chaperoning policy, whereas Jones et al. [66] showed that 95 % of general practitioners surveyed in Melbourne, Australia, had never or only occasionally used a chaperone. A survey of lead clinicians in Emergency Departments in the UK, reported that less than 4 % of departments had a formal chaperoning policy [67]. In that study, it was concerning, that about a quarter of respondents reported incidents of complaints about inappropriate examination by doctors. Sinha et al. [68] evaluated the attitudes of patients in breast examination. They reported that most patients consider the offer, or use, of a chaperone as a sign of respect. Patients did not consider having a chaperone as harming the patient-doctor relationship, breaching confidentiality, or causing embarrassment.

Consider having a chaperone present in your consultations, or examinations of patients, as a way of protecting your patients but also looking after yourself too. A chaperone may help protect you against false allegations of misconduct, or inappropriate behaviour. Such allegations may not be the result of malaise, but may arise due to poor communication, patient's misunderstanding as to what the examination involves, or patient's mental health problems.

Being rushed for time, staff shortages, or lack of resources, are not justifiable reasons for not using a chaperone. Consider the stress and impact upon yourself, if allegations were to happen. Consider the time and effort you would have to put in for your defence.

What ever your sex, or the patient's sex, consider a chaperone for most consultations and examinations. It helps protect both the patient and yourself. Use an independent, third party chaperone, someone who understands what medical examinations involve rather than simply a patient's friend, relative or medical administrator. Document the offer and presence of a chaperone, but note that "merely offering a chaperone does not protect either the patient or the doctor" [69].

Join a Union

The 40-hour work week, the minimum wage, family leave, health insurance, social security, medicare, retirement plans. The cornerstones of the middle-class security all bear the union label

Barack Obama [1]

You may turn up to work with great enthusiasm, best intentions, put all effort and hard work, try and improve the service, provide high quality care, or give lots of unpaid time, but your management, co-workers or boss may not appreciate it. They may decide to cut your pay, increase your working hours, introduce antisocial working. You may be picked on, targeted, harassed. You may be signing a contract with an employer but you don't understand the fine print, the legal language.

The government may introduce changes to your pension scheme, remuneration, or holiday allowance. Jobs may be cut, redundancies made. You may be self employed but regulations and restrictions are mounting. You may be in a training program, and the training may be shortened, experience diluted. You may need advice about ethical decisions, or simply a shoulder to cry on.

Organised groups have a bigger say, more power, are more resistant to pressure. It may be better not to fight the cause alone. Unions may be able to give you legal advice, truly confirm your rights and obligations, join you in employment or other dispute meetings, negotiate terms and conditions, take industrial action. Do not wait until problems arise, join a supporting group or two.

The following are some of the factors you may consider in choosing which group to join:

- The size of the union's membership.
- The degree of representation of the union amongst other healthcare workers in your workplace.
- Its reputation for giving easy access for prompt advice.
- Its reputation in providing representation in person, in workplace disputes.
- Whether it would support you with legal aid, in dealing with disputes.

Stay Positive

Keep your face to the sunshine and you cannot see a shadow

Helen Keller [1]

Medicine, like many other professions, may have its ups and downs. There may be times when you feel despair, when the physical, or emotional pressures take their toll. There may be times when the workload, tiredness, and fatigue are mounting. There may be times when things seem gloomy, when the future is uncertain, when long term plans are difficult to make. There may be times when you may have to keep trying to pass that vital exam, when you may have to keep searching for that, well sought after, post. There may be times when you may have to, once more, relocate around the country for that important job, or even migrate for a better future.

There may be times when you question the red tape, the regulations, the unfair cover of the profession by the media, the lack of mutual courtesy and respect, the blurring of roles and titles.

It may be easy to get cynical, adopt a pessimistic approach, and just go with the general bleak mood. However, even in days of despair, at times of crises, keep a positive outlook. Being positive may be essential to pull not only yourself, but also, all those around you, through the challenges faced. Others may look at you for strength and support.

Stay positive. Medicine is a great profession. Becoming a doctor is a great achievement, an accomplishment to be proud of. In difficult times, reflect back on what you attained, and what you went through, to reach where you are. Reflect back on the great enthusiasm of the new start, the goals you met through hard work and perseverance, the skills you gained through enthusiasm and determination. Remind yourself of the situations where you improved someone's life, made someone feel so much better, when you comforted and reassured others.

Stay positive and stick to your principles. Ensure that all you do is your choice. Ensure that all you do, you are comfortable with.

References

1. Brainyquote. http://www.brainyquote.com. Accessed on 26 Sept 2014
2. Volkswagen turns off Blackberry email after work hours. BBC News technology. http://www.bbc.co.uk/news/technology. Accessed on 26 Sept 2014
3. Email obsession 'will impact Christmas holidays. BBC News technology. http://www.bbc.co.uk/news/technology. Accessed on 26 Sept 2014
4. Mangan L. When the French clock off at 6pm, they really mean it. The Guardian, 2014. http://www.theguardian.com. Accessed on 26 Sept 2014
5. Winston CP, Sallis JF, Swartz MD, Hoelscher DM, Peskin MF. Reliability of the hospital nutrition environment scan for cafeterias, vending machines, and gift shops. J Acad Nutr Diet. 2013;113(8):1069–75.
6. Winston CP, Sallis JF, Swartz MD, Hoelscher DM, Peskin MF. Consumer nutrition environments of hospitals: an exploratory analysis using the hospital nutrition environment scan for cafeterias, vending machines, and gift shops, 2012. Prev Chron Dis. 2013;10:E110.
7. Lederer A, Toner C, Krepp EM, Curtis CJ. Understanding hospital cafeterias: results from cafeteria manager interviews. J Publ Health Manag Pract. 2014;20(1 Suppl 1):S50–3.
8. McDermott N. Weight's up doc: fat medics ordered to slim by NHS chief. The Sun, 2014. http://www.thesun.co.uk. Accessed on 26 Sept 2014
9. Horrocks N, Pounder R, RCP Working Group. Working the night shift: preparation, survival and recovery – a guide for junior doctors. Clin Med. 2006;6(1):61–7.
10. Tewari A, Soliz J, Billota F, Garg S, Singh H. Does our sleep debt affect patients' safety? Indian J Anaesth. 2011;55(1):12–7.
11. Parthasarathy S. Sleep and the medical profession. Curr Opin Pulm Med. 2005;11(6):507–12.
12. Rauchenzauner M, Ernst F, Hintringer F, Ulmer H, Ebenbichler CF, Kasseroler MT, Joannidis M. Arrhythmias and increased neuro-endocrine stress response during physicians' night shifts: a randomized cross-over trial. Eur Heart J. 2009;30(21):2606–13.
13. Belayachi J, Benjelloun O, Madani N, Abidi K, Dendane T, Zeggwagh AA, Abouqal R. Self-perceived sleepiness in emergency training physicians: prevalence and relationship with quality of life. J Occup Med Toxicol. 2013;8(1):24. doi:10.1186/1745-6673-8-24.
14. Samkoff JS, Jacques CH. A review of studies concerning effects of sleep deprivation and fatigue on residents' performance. Acad Med. 1991;66:687–93.
15. Frese M, Okonek KA. Reasons to leave shiftwork and psychological and psychosomatic complaints of former shiftworkers. J Appl Psychol. 1984;69:509–14.
16. Kawachi I, Colditz GA, Stampfer MJ, Willett WC, Manson JE, Speizer FE, Hennekens CH. Prospective study of shift work and risk of coronary heart disease in women. Circulation. 1995;92:3178–82.
17. Brennan TA, Zinner MJ. Residents' work hours: a wakeup call? Int J Qual Health Care. 2003;15:107–8.
18. Howard SK, Gaba DM, Rosekind MR, Zarcone VP. The risks and implications of excessive daytime sleepiness in resident physicians. Acad Med. 2002;77:1019–25.
19. Papp KK, Stoller EP, Sage P, Aikens JE, Owens J, Avidan A, Phillips B, Rosen R, Strohl KP. The effects of sleep loss and fatigue on resident physicians: a multi-institutional, mixed method study. Acad Med. 2004;79:394–406.
20. Arnedt JT, Owens J, Crouch M, Stahl J, Carskadon MA. Neurobehavioral performance of residents after heavy night calls after alcohol ingestion. JAMA. 2005;294:1025–33.
21. Fujino Y, Iso H, Tamakoshi A, Inaba Y, Koizumi A, Kubo T, Yoshimura T. A prospective cohort study of shift work and risk of ischemic heart disease in Japanese male workers. Am J Epidemiol. 2006;164:128–35.
22. Furlan R, Barbic F, Piazza S, Tinelli M, Seghizzi P, Malliani A. Modifications of cardiac autonomic profile associated with a shift schedule of work. Circulation. 2000;102:1912–6.
23. Knutsson A, Boggild H. Shiftwork and cardiovascular disease: review of disease mechanisms. Rev Environ Health. 2000;15:359–72.

24. Adams SL, Roxe DM, Weiss J, Zhang F, Rosenthal JE. Ambulatory blood pressure and Holter monitoring of emergency physicians before, during, and after a night shift. Acad Emerg Med. 1998;5:871–7.

25. Theorell T, Akerstedt T. Day and night work: changes in cholesterol, uric acid, glucose and potassium in serum and in circadian patterns of urinary catecholamine excretion. A longitudinal cross-over study of railway workers. Acta Med Scand. 1976;200:47–53.

26. Baldwin Jr DC, Daugherty SR. Sleep deprivation and fatigue in residency training: results of a national survey of first- and second-year residents. Sleep. 2004;27(2):217–23.

27. Department of Health. Strategy statement on physical activity. London: Department of Health; 1996.

28. Department of Health. More people, more active, more often. London: Department of Health; 1996.

29. Gupta K, Fan L. Doctors: fighting fit or couch potatoes? Brit J Sports Med. 2009;43:153–4.

30. Leventer-Roberts M, Zonfrillo MR, Yu S, Dziura JD, Spiro DM. Overweight physicians during residency: a cross-sectional and longitudinal study. J Grad Med Educ. 2013;5(3):405–11.

31. O'Cathail M, O'Callaghan M. A profile of hospital consultants: the health practices of a cohort of medical professionals. Ir Med J. 2013;106(5):134–6.

32. Pardo A, McKenna J, Mitjans A, Camps B, Aranda-García S, Garcia-Gil J, Violan M. Physical activity level and lifestyle-related risk factors from catalan physicians. J Phys Act Health. 2014;11(5):922–9.

33. AlAteeq MA, AlArawi SM. Healthy lifestyle among primary health care professionals. Saudi Med J. 2014;35(5):488–94.

34. Waseem M, Kornberg RJ. A sedentary job? Measuring the physical activity of emergency medicine residents. J Emerg Med. 2013;44(1):204–8.

35. Le Masurier GC, Sidman CL, Corbin CB. Accumulating 10,000 steps: does this meet current physical activity guidelines? Res Q Exerc Sport. 2003;74:389–94.

36. Pate RR, Pratt M, Blair SN, Haskell WL, Macera CA, Bouchard C, Buchner D, Ettinger W, Heath GW, King AC. Physical activity and public health. A recommendation from the Centers for Disease Control and Prevention and the American College of Sports Medicine. JAMA. 1995;273:402–7.

37. U.S. Department of Health and Human Services. Physical activity and health: a report of the Surgeon General. Atlanta: U.S. Department of Health and Human Services, Centers for Disease Control and Prevention, National Center for Chronic Disease Prevention and Health Promotion; 1996.

38. ER/NBC. http://www.nbc.com/er. Accessed on 26 Sept 2014

39. Weight CJ, Sellon JL, Lessard-Anderson CR, Shanafelt TD, Olsen KD, Laskowski ER. Physical activity, quality of life, and burnout among physician trainees: the effect of a team-based, incentivized exercise program. Mayo Clin Proc. 2013;88(12):1435–42.

40. Bruguera M, Gurí J, Arteman A, Grau Valldosera J, Carbonell J. Doctors taking care of their own health. Results of a postal survey. Med Clin (Barc). 2001;117(13):492–4.

41. Chen JY, Tse EY, Lam TP, Li DK, Chao DV, Kwan CW. Doctors' personal health care choices: a cross-sectional survey in a mixed public/private setting. BMC Public Health. 2008;8:183.

42. Pullen D, Lonie CE, Lyle DM, Cam DE, Doughty MV. Medical care of doctors. Med J Aust. 1995;162(9):481, 484.

43. Ghodse H. Doctors and their health — who heals the healers? In: Ghodse H, Mann S, Johnson P, editors. Doctors and their health. Sutton: Reed Healthcare Limited; 2000.

44. Hawton K, Clements A, Sakarovitch C, et al. Suicide in doctors: a study of risk according to gender, seniority and specialty in medical practitioners in England and Wales, 1979–1995. J Epidemiol Community Health. 2001;55:296–300.

45. Shanafelt TD, Balch CM, Dyrbye L, Bechamps G, Russell T, Satele D, Rummans T, Swartz K, Novotny PJ, Sloan J, Oreskovich MR. Special report: suicidal ideation among American surgeons. Arch Surg. 2011;146(1):54–62.

46. McKevitt C, Morgan M, Dundas R, Holland WW. Sickness absence and 'working through' illness: a comparison of two professional groups. J Public Health Med. 1997;19(3):295–300.

47. Perkin MR, Higton A, Witcomb M. Do junior doctors take sick leave? Occup Environ Med. 2003;60(9):699–700.
48. Yerkes RM, Dodson JD. The relation of strength of stimulus to rapidity of habit-formation. J Comp Neurol Psychol. 1908;18:459–82.
49. Anderson CR. Coping behaviors as intervening mechanisms in the inverted-U stress-performance relationship. J Appl Psychol. 1976;61(7):30–4.
50. Diamond DM, Campbell AM, Park CR, Halonen J, Zoladz PR. The temporal dynamics model of emotional memory processing: a synthesis on the neurobiological basis of stress-induced amnesia, flashbulb and traumatic memories, and the Yerkes-Dodson law. Neural Plast. 2007;2007:60803.
51. Lam TP, Wong JG, Ip MS, Lam KF, Pang SL. Psychological well-being of interns in Hong Kong: what causes them stress and what helps them. Med Teach. 2010;32(3):e120–6.
52. Maslach C, Schaufeli WB, Leiter MP. Job burnout. Annu Rev Psychol. 2001;52:397–422.
53. Maslach C, Jackson SE. The measurement of experienced burnout. J Occup Behav. 1981;2:99–113.
54. Leung J, Rioseco P, Munro P. Stress, satisfaction and burnout amongst Australian and New Zealand radiation oncologists. J Med Imaging Radiat Oncol. 2014. doi:10.1111/1754-9485.
55. Streu R, Hansen J, Abrahamse P, Alderman AK. Professional burnout among US plastic surgeons: results of a national survey. Ann Plast Surg. 2014;72(3):346–50.
56. van Vendeloo SN, Brand PL, Verheyen CC. Burnout and quality of life among orthopaedic trainees in a modern educational programme: importance of the learning climate. Bone Joint J. 2014;96-B(8):1133–8.
57. Shanafelt TD, Balch CM, Bechamps GJ, Russell T, Dyrbye L, Satele D, Collicott P, Novotny PJ, Sloan J, Freischlag JA. Burnout and career satisfaction among American surgeons. Ann Surg. 2009;250(3):463–71.
58. Castelo-Branco C, Figueras F, Eixarch E, Quereda F, Cancelo MJ, González S, Balasch J. Stress symptoms and burnout in obstetric and gynaecology residents. BJOG. 2007;114(1):94–8.
59. Shanafelt TD, Boone S, Tan L, Dyrbye LN, Sotile W, Satele D, West CP, Sloan J, Oreskovich MR. Burnout and satisfaction with work-life balance among US physicians relative to the general US population. Arch Intern Med. 2012;172(18):1377–85.
60. Aldrees TM, Aleissa S, Zamakhshary M, Badri M, Sadat-Ali M. Physician well-being: prevalence of burnout and associated risk factors in a tertiary hospital, Riyadh, Saudi Arabia. Ann Saudi Med. 2013;33(5):451–6.
61. Leiter MP, Maslach C. Six areas of worklife: a model of the organizational context of burnout. J Health Hum Serv Adm. 1999;21(4):472–89.
62. Sagan C. Pale blue dot. 1994. Planetary Society. http://www.planetary.org/explore/space-topics/earth/pale-blue-dot.html. Accessed on 27 Sept 2014
63. Wazana A. Physicians and the Pharmaceutical Industry: is a gift ever just a gift? J Am Med Assoc. 2000;283:373–80.
64. Seabury S, Chandra A, Lakdawalla D, Jena AB. Defense costs of medical malpractice claims. N Engl J Med. 2012;366(14):1354–6.
65. Rosenthal J, Rymer J, Jones R, Haldane S, Cohen S, Bartholomew J. Chaperones for intimate examinations: cross sectional survey of attitudes and practices of general practitioners. BMJ. 2005;330(7485):234–5.
66. Jones K, Biezen R, Beovich B, van Hecke O. Chaperones for intimate examinations in family medicine: findings from a pilot study in Melbourne, Australia. Med Sci Law. 2014.
67. Loizides S, Kallis A, Oswal A, Georgiou P, Kallis G, Gavalas M. Chaperone policy in accident and emergency departments: a national survey. J Eval Clin Pract. 2010;16(1):107–10.
68. Sinha S, De A, Williams RJ, Vaughan-Williams E. Use of a chaperone during breast examination: the attitude and practice of consultant breast surgeons in the United Kingdom. Scott Med J. 2010;55(1):24–6.
69. Conway S, Harvey I. Use and offering of chaperones by general practitioners: postal questionnaire survey in Norfolk. BMJ. 2005;330:235–6.

Index

© Springer International Publishing Switzerland 2015
C. Panayiotou Charalambous, *Career Skills for Doctors*,
DOI 10.1007/978-3-319-13479-6